THE GIFTS BENEATH YOUR ANXIETY

THE
GIFTS BENEATH
YOUR ANXIETY

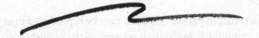

Simple Spiritual Tools to Find Peace, Awaken
the Power Within, and Heal Your Life

Pat Longo

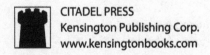

CITADEL PRESS
Kensington Publishing Corp.
www.kensingtonbooks.com

CITADEL PRESS BOOKS are published by

Kensington Publishing Corp.
119 West 40th Street
New York, NY 10018

All Kensington titles, imprints, and distributed lines are available at special quantity discounts for bulk purchases for sales promotions, premiums, fund-raising, educational, or institutional use. Special book excerpts or customized printings can also be created to fit specific needs. For details, write or phone the office of the Kensington sales manager: Kensington Publishing Corp., 119 West 40th Street, New York, NY 10018, attn: Sales Department; phone 1-800-221-2647.

CITADEL PRESS and the Citadel logo are Reg. U.S. Pat. & TM Off.

ISBN-13: 978-0-8065-3943-0
ISBN-10: 0-8065-3943-7

First hardcover printing: September 2019

10 9 8 7 6 5 4 3 2 1

Printed in the United States of America

Library of Congress Control Number: TK

Electronic edition:

ISBN-13: 978-0-8065-3945-4 (e-book)
ISBN-10: 0-8065-3945-3 (e-book)

Contents

Introduction

"YOU'RE A WHAT?" THIS IS the question, along with many others, that I often receive when I tell people I'm a spiritual healer and teacher. They seem taken aback that I appear to be a "regular" person and am not sporting horns and a tail and waving around dead chickens. But no one was more surprised than I was when, over twenty years ago, I discovered I had healing hands. I was just your everyday forty-something frantically busy wife, homemaker, soccer mom of five (including twins!), and dedicated chauffeur of said children when I decided I needed to stop the chaos and do something for me. I ultimately joined a spiritual awareness class, and one day shortly thereafter, out of the blue, felt my hands begin to heat up. They felt like they were on fire. I had no idea why. Nor did I have any idea that what would transpire next would be, to my complete shock and bewilderment, the beginning of my unexpected journey as a spiritual healer.

Over time I have found that, for me, healing is the process of bringing one's whole self into balance and opening the pathway for one to be fully realized in all he or she is meant to be. As a spiritual healer, I work through my spiritual connection and intention to bring God's love, light, and healing energy through me, through my hands (whether in person or long distance), and into the individual(s) in need of healing. Over time, I have also come to understand that it is essential for people to learn how to participate in their own healing and maintenance of their health as part of their day-to-day lives.

Having been a spiritual healer and teacher for more than two decades, I have been blessed to have had the opportunity to help thousands of individuals in need of healing from all types of conditions, ranging from heartache to physical injury, infection, autoimmune disease, neuromuscular disease, and cancer. But there has been one condition that has presented in my practice over and over again with astounding frequency. Countless men, women, and children have come to me suffering with unexplained anxiety. Again and again, they have described to me feelings of anxiety and related symptoms such as unexplained racing heart, panic attacks, nausea, digestive issues, headache, feelings of sadness and depression, a sense of being overwhelmed by other people's moods and feelings, and even phobias of leaving the house, being around crowds or other people, or being alone (especially at night). For many individuals, this anxiety is chronic and can persist even after consulting with their physicians and therapists.

While I am saddened to know that so many people are suffering with these symptoms, I have great hope for their future. You see, we know that chronic anxiety can be caused by a number of contributors including genetic and environmental factors. But what if there were another, hidden potential cause of anxiety—one that is related to our nature as spiritual beings and the spiritual gifts that we possess? After seeing so many clients with unexplained chronic anxiety, this is exactly what I have found. The good news is, I have also found that a spiritual approach to healing and care can be effective in alleviating this type of anxiety, sometimes quite quickly! I have seen this approach work for thousands of individuals, many of whom not only experienced relief from their anxiety, but also began to discover and embrace the spiritual gifts they never knew they had.

You see, each of us is a soul, or spiritual being, who is here on earth to have the experience of being human. Because of our spiritual nature, each of us has spiritual needs and spiritual gifts to recognize, protect, and develop and use for our own and the greater good. I believe our *intuition* is a fundamental spiritual gift that, as spiritual beings, we all possess. I think of our intuition as a sensing, knowing, feeling, or otherwise perceiving that is derived not through our human experience or the normal range of our five physical senses, but through our connection to our own spiritual selves and to God and the Universe around us. We often experience our intuition as that still, small voice inside of us, or that inner feeling, that serves to guide, teach, and protect us. Have you ever had a gut feeling? Or met someone new and felt that brick-wall "no" sensation in your stomach? Have you ever thought of a person you hadn't heard from in years, only to have tthem call a few minutes later? Or maybe you've felt the hair on the back of your neck stand up, only to turn and find that someone was watching you. The gift of intuition resides in all of us. I further believe that our intuition can also manifest asmore specific spiritual gifts like those sometimes referred to as psychic ability, mediumship, and spiritual healing. In my experience, very few people are aware of having these gifts and are in complete disbelief at the suggestion that they may. Some may think it's a little too *out there*, but I find it, well, natural. We are indeed all spiritual beings and we all have spiritual selves, needs, and gifts.

This is why, when caring for our health and well-being, it's important to take care of our whole selves—the physical, emotional, mental, and spiritual parts of us. I believe wholeheartedly that our physicians, therapists, nurses, and other healthcare professionals are essential in helping us to maintain our health. At the same time, while we work with our health professionals to care for our physical and mental selves, we must also ensure that our spiritual self receives the care and attention it needs. This means recognizing that we are spiritual beings and making the time in our busy lives to connect with our spiritual selves. This can be done by spending quiet time in nature, participating in meditation exercises, visiting a place of worship, or any number of other ways. It means making a point to listen to our intuition, to that still small voice inside, and let it guide us. It means finding what feeds our spirit and honoring ourselves by making time for those things. And finally, based on my findings, it means using very simple spiritual tools and exercises in our daily lives that can help us to protect, nourish, and care for our spiritual selves and energy. When we care for our whole selves, this keeps us in balance, maintains the flow of our energy, and helps us to live in a state of health and healing. It also opens the door for us to become aware of and recognize our spiritual gifts. When we don't take care of our spiritual selves, like any other part of ourselves, I believe this balance can be disrupted and symptoms and illness can develop as a result. And for those with exceptionally strong intuitive abilities, or spiritual gifts, a lack of awareness, protection, and care can lead to—you guessed it—anxiety and other related symptoms.

Spiritual care is important for everyone, and it is especially essential for people whom I would call *empaths*. Over the years, I have found that the majority of my clients suffering with unexplained anxiety were by their nature empaths—individuals who possess a heightened sensitivity to the energy around them and, I believe, a heightened sense of intuition. Overall, empaths are highly sensitive people and they may experience this sensitivity in a number of ways. In terms of physical stimuli, empaths can have a heightened sensitivity to one or more stimuli such as certain lighting, sounds, smells, tastes, or even touch. For example, they may need to wear sunglasses more frequently or get headaches from fluorescent lighting or certain fragrances. Or they may get overwhelmed by too much stimuli coming at them all at once.

This sensitivity also extends beyond the physical five senses. I often refer to empaths as energy sponges. Everything is made of energy, from people to animals, plants, nature, places, and objects. Our thoughts, feelings, and intentions also are made of energy. Since we are all made of energy and all are interconnected, every one of us perceives, receives, and transmits energy every single day. While we all have the intuitive ability to sense energy beyond the normal range of our five senses, empaths perceive and receive energy in the extreme. For example, many people could walk into a room and feel a general sense of enthusiasm, grief, anger, or tension so thick that "you could cut it with a knife." But I believe empaths feel this energy more strongly and often actually absorb, take on, and experience the energy as their own. It's for this reason that many empaths prefer to avoid, or even have phobias of, large groups or gatherings, such as work, school, or social events. Imagine going to school or work and feeling not only your own thoughts and emotions, but those of everyone and everything around you—happiness, sadness, grief, guilt, shame, jealousy, anger, worry, fear, good intentions, ill intentions. For many empaths, this is what everyday life is like. My goodness, this could give anyone anxiety! Indeed, for an empath who is not aware of this heightened sensitivity and is not able to take the preventive measures needed to protect him- or herself, the absorption of these energies can lead to the development of extreme anxiety and, sometimes, other symptoms and conditions.

So I believe at least part of an empath's heightened ability to sense, feel, or otherwise perceive the energies around them is being mediated by a heightened gift of intuition. Now imagine that this heightened intuitive ability is allowing them to perceive not only the energies of the people, animals, and places around them, but also those of beings in the spirit world. Again, I believe we all have this intuitive ability, but I have found that empaths are highly likely to have an exceptionally strong ability in this area. Our intuition can manifest as a number of strong spiritual gifts—like psychic, mediumship, or spiritual healing abilities. However, I have found (so far) that my empath clients who have had anxiety are more likely to possess exceptionally strong psychic or mediumship gifts, meaning the ability to receive information from the Universe or spirit world or communicate directly with beings who are in spirit form. Unfortunately, very few know they have these abilities when they first come to see me for anxiety! When asked, some of my clients and students, for example, would report that they had been seeing, hearing, and feeling things that other people didn't from the time they were small children but did not understand what was happening. Others said they were afraid of this part of themselves, believing that they were crazy or even evil. Most people were completely unaware of these gifts or dismissed their experiences as their imagination or as random thoughts that just came and went. They had in effect tried to ignore, dismiss, compartmentalize, or otherwise push down these experiences and therefore push down the energy from the spirit world that was coming in with them. But when a communication is not recognized or received, it can often continue to come and come and come. And for people who ignore or bottle it up, this energy inevitably bubbles its way to the surface, erupting in the form of anxiety and other symptoms. Unable to recognize and accept this spiritual part of themselves, these beautiful souls were fighting their own truth, their own destinies, and it was making them sick.

Now I know you may be thinking—there's no way, this is crazy, this is not me, I don't have anything like this happening to me. Let me just tell you this is exactly what most of my clients said! But once they tried a few simple spiritual exercises to help them, they realized that they were in fact experiencing spiritually based anxiety—and that they didn't have to live like this anymore.

The good news is, if you suffer from spiritually based anxiety and other empath-related symptoms, you don't have to live like this either. Using the simple steps and tools that I employ in my spiritual healing sessions—designed to restore and maintain balance to the spiritual, mental, emotional, and physical bodies—I have seen countless individuals be freed from the prison of anxiety and associated symptoms. With this same spiritual healing approach, you too can learn to heal and to protect yourself and your energy. And as you heal and learn to maintain this more balanced state, you will also learn how to begin to discover and accept your own gift of intuition. In turn, as you start to open to and love this part of yourself, you will find even more healing, more balance, and further alleviation of anxiety and other related symptoms.

Before we begin, I just want to talk about some of the terminology I will use throughout the book. I often will refer to my faith in and connection with God. This is my personal belief. If you believe differently, that's okay. You just need to be open to connecting with your spiritual self and with a higher power or consciousness of goodness that is greater than yourself. I call this God. You can call it "The Universe," "The Source," "Yahweh," "Allah," "Jehovah," "The Divine," "the consciousness of love and light," or whatever term works for you. Similarly, in reference to health and healing, I refer to our "whole selves" as inclusive of all the parts of ourselves, meaning our spiritual, mental, emotional, and physical "selves" or "bodies." In turn, I use the hyphenated term "dis-ease" to refer to any block, disruption, or disturbance in the balance and wellness of our four selves or bodies. This is inclusive of symptoms, conditions, and illness, which can both contribute to and manifest as a result of this disturbance. Finally, you do not have to agree with every single thing I say in the book to benefit from it. I encourage you to assess the information for yourself and use what resonates for you. The most important thing is that, whatever you do, you set your intention to do it "for the highest good."

It is my intention with this book to walk you through the process of spiritual healing. I want to teach you how to heal, maintain your health and well-being, and discover your own gift of intuition as part of that healing. I encourage you to use the book as your personal tool kit, as a guide in your journey to love and heal your whole self. As we turn the next pages together, you will find guidance and simple tools to help you protect yourself spiritually; identify and address areas in need of balance and healing; open to your spiritual gifts; and eliminate the spiritual causes of anxiety and other suffering in your life. In doing so, you will find healing, balance, and the peace and fulfillment that comes only with accepting, realizing, and living your own truth. And then, you will be free.

CHAPTER 1

Are You an Empath?

*O*VER MY MORE THAN TWENTY years as a spiritual healer and teacher, many of my clients and students who were suffering with unexplained anxiety, panic attacks, irrational fears, phobias, and related symptoms would turn out to be empaths. For some, their symptoms had escalated to the point that they had become a detriment to their quality of life, a veritable prison, and yet a cause for their condition could not be found. The good news is that, when I began to discover that these individuals were empaths—and that their anxiety was related to their having a heightened sensitivity to the energy around them and, I believe, a heightened sense of intuition—I found that there were some very simple exercises that could help them.

So what is an empath—and how do you know if you are one? Most empaths I have met did not know they were empaths and certainly had no idea they might be harboring any type of special intuitive gift. This was also true for me. In fact, it was only in learning how to take time for myself, to listen to and honor myself, that I ultimately discovered my own gift as a spiritual healer. Later, in my work as a healer, I discovered that I had been an empath all along. And, while I never had anxiety myself, I began to see the connection between empaths, spiritual energy, and anxiety revealed in my clients and students.

My Story:
Listening to the Still Small Voice Within

For as long as I can remember, I believed my soul's purpose was to be a wife, mother, and grandmother. It wasn't until my mid-forties that I discovered I also was called to be a spiritual healer and teacher.

As a young wife and mother, I felt completely fulfilled in the beautiful life I had, but I always felt a little something tugging at my core, a deep-down desire. I knew there was something more, but I just didn't know what that was back then. I didn't have any obvious problems or issues that were bothering me. I just felt that something was missing.

As a child and young adult I had suffered with various illnesses, including asthma, allergies, eczema, severe migraines, sinus infections, irritable bowel syndrome, bronchitis, several bouts of pneumonia, and others. I seemed to come down with *everything*. I was also allergic to many medications and, at some point, developed an allergy to fragrances. The smell alone of a strong perfume, lotion, or soap could send me into anaphylaxis. While I seemed to be sick more frequently than the average child, my life overall had been happy and, well... normal.

I was born and raised by wonderful parents, as part of a large Catholic family on Long Island. I am the second-born of six children and have strong relationships with my five siblings. I married the love of my life, Vinny, in 1968. We were both very young, eighteen and nineteen years old. Over the next six years, we proceeded to have five beautiful children, completing our family in 1975 with a set of twin boys. Needless to say, my life became a little chaotic during this time.

As the years flew by, I dedicated my time and attention to our family and its myriad of activities. I became involved in the PTA of our children's public elementary school and volunteered as the teacher for the weekly fourth-grade religion class at our local Catholic school. I was on the board of our neighborhood civic association and was the den mother of our sons' Cub Scout troop. The girls belonged to a Brownie troop and attended dance school, and the boys played on multiple sports teams. My husband worked long hours and often traveled with his job. Much of the time I was on my own and, as many parents know, a good deal of my effort was spent, you guessed it, schlepping. I loved my family and friends more than anything, but by the time I hit my late thirties, I didn't know whether I was coming or going. I gave no thought to my own wants or needs and had completely lost myself.

All of this came to a screeching halt the night of one fateful Tupperware party. It was one home-improvement event too many. A friend had invited me to her house for the occasion and, although I was exhausted, I wanted to show my support and agreed to attend. I have nothing against Tupperware or parties, I had attended dozens, but this happened to be the one where I hit the wall—my wall. The party was lovely, but I quite simply had not wanted to be there.

When the event finished, I came home, walked into the living room, looked at my husband, and proclaimed, "I'm done.

I'm everybody's everything and I don't know where I begin or where I end." He looked at me as though I had lost my mind. Perhaps I had, just for a few minutes. Yet, for me, this was a moment of unmistakable clarity. The next day, to the dismay of family and friends, I proceeded to resign from many of my extracurricular activities. I finished out my terms and fulfilled all of my commitments, but gave notices to the PTA, civic association, Cub Scouts, and religion class that I would not be renewing those commitments going forward. In their place, I started taking adult tap-dancing lessons and joined a bowling league. I had finally decided that I was important too. I needed to honor and love myself, by putting me first for a change. I happily maintained my obligations to my family, still did the necessary schlepping, but I no longer felt pulled in twenty directions at once. And two nights a week, I was doing something just for me.

As a result of this shift in my energy, an astonishing thing happened. When I began saying no to some of the countless activities and invitations coming my way, my life became more balanced and I began to hear that still small voice inside, whispering that there was something more. This time, I listened. I felt a need to find the answer to what was tugging at my core. Instead of my usual romance novels, I began to read spiritual books, consuming them by the dozens.

At the same time I was enjoying this spiritual awakening, I also started to experience physical pain and swelling in my joints. The symptoms first hit in 1987 when my twin boys' soccer team held a leaf-raking campaign to raise funds for a European tournament. Of course, the parents were the ones doing the raking, and I noticed a severe aching in my elbow at that time. The pain continued for months and was initially diagnosed as tennis elbow. Over time, I developed this same pain in multiple joints, all on the right side of my body. It moved to my ankle, then to my shoulder, and after a few years finally landed in my hip. The hip pain became so severe that I had difficulty sleeping at night. Several years after its onset, the condition was diagnosed by a rheumatologist as psoriatic arthritis. Although there was treatment available, I found it to be too expensive and too toxic to tolerate.

While in the process of trying to find other treatment options for the arthritic condition, I received even more distressing news. My mother had been diagnosed with inoperable breast cancer that had metastasized to her bones. Her prognosis was poor. Even with the recommended treatment regimen, the doctor advised us that she did not expect my mother to live for much more than a year. Like many others who have faced a cancer diagnosis, my family was absolutely panicked. Little did I know that in the midst of these health crises, when things seemed darkest, a whole new world was getting ready to open up before me.

Within a few weeks of my mother's diagnosis, I found myself sitting with a psychic. He immediately began giving me highly accurate messages, regarding "a mother figure" about whom I was worried and incredible details about her diagnosis and poor prognosis. He also directed me to a "spiritual healer" who allegedly had some success with treating persons diagnosed with cancer. While skeptical, we were desperate and I figured we had nothing to lose. I made an appointment and took my mother to see the healer the following day. Afterward, my mother seemed like a different person. Sitting in the car outside, she told me that the healer had performed an energy healing on her—and also had asked what was "eating her up" inside. In fact, my mother said there *had* been something that had been bothering her for years. Now instead of hanging on to this emotional pain, she had let it go. She had a new peace, a lightness about her. After that one healing session, my mother began to feel better. She also underwent the recommended chemo for a while and then hormone therapy, even though it was not expected to provide much benefit. Subsequent blood tests revealed that my mother's tumor markers had dropped and scans showed the cancer had stopped growing. This effect was sustained for the next fifteen years, with the cancer in relative stagnation, until my mother died of natural causes at age eighty-four. (My father had passed away the year before, and she simply did not wish to be here without him.)

This miraculous turn of events was not only a God-send for my mother and our family, but it was also a spiritual ah-hah moment for me. I reflected back on my twenties, when I would see the occasional psychic at a psychic fair. I had viewed this as entertainment, not something to be taken seriously. Every now and then, however, I would meet a psychic who connected with me, providing highly detailed and accurate information. I would wonder how he or she could know these things. Several of these individuals had also told me I was a healer. Now *that* I thought was crazy. I had no idea what they were talking about. I thought perhaps they were suggesting that I become a doctor or nurse, but I had five children and no budget for medical or nursing school. I didn't know what it meant to be a healer and dismissed it completely, until this experience with my mother. The word "healer" had suddenly become something real to me. Within days of my mother's appointment, the Universe would lead me right to the door that would change my life.

On a Saturday afternoon, as I was getting ready to pull out of my driveway, our youngest son Daniel ran out to the car to show me an advertisement in a local paper. He was a teenager at the time, and this was highly unusual behavior for him. The ad was promoting an event to be held at a nearby hotel, featur-

ing spiritual medium James Van Praagh. Given my recent experience, this event was suddenly of great interest to me. I had
developed a voracious appetite for any information that could
aid me in my quest for all things spiritual. When I called to pur-
chase tickets, the woman on the phone also directed me to a
teacher in my area who was offering a class focused on spiritual awareness. The teacher's name was Holly Chalnick, and
she was the answer to my prayers.

I started Holly's class and enjoyed it tremendously. I
learned how to use meditation to connect with my spiritual
self; to balance, protect, and ground myself; and to use various
methods and techniques to tap into and develop my intuition.
However, within three weeks, something disconcerting oc-
curred. My hands inexplicably began to heat up. They felt like
red-hot poker irons. I had no idea what was causing this uncomfortable sensation. Was I in menopause? Was I having hot
flashes in my hands? I was concerned enough to mention this
phenomenon to Holly, who seemed to be interested but not
alarmed. Then one day in class, she instructed me to place my
hand on the woman next to me who had been experiencing
residual joint pain from an old car accident. "What—why
would I do that?!" I thought to myself. But I complied and,
with the woman's permission, I put my hand on her leg.
Within a few short minutes, she reported that her pain had
vanished. My head was spinning with thoughts of how this
could be. Because Holly's expertise was focused on using our
intuition as a form of connection and communication more
than on healing, she encouraged me to continue to take her
class while also exploring other sources of information on
spiritual healing specifically. I soon found myself at the local
library, searching for books on hands-on healing, anything I
could find to help explain this incident. Back then, I didn't
even know where to look. I ended up trying the psychology

and religion sections. I began reading on spirituality, intuition, energy, and manifestation. I read hundreds of books, practically swallowing them whole.

As I combed the literature for more information to help explain or instruct me in spiritual or hands-on healing, my gift continued to develop. I wasn't ready to share this newfound interest with anyone quite yet, but I started quietly (and covertly) practicing on my siblings and children. In doing so, I inadvertently began taking on their physical symptoms, which baffled me. This happened one night when my sisters Eileen and Carol were relaxing in the hot tub at a friend's house. Everyone has always loved my massages, so when Eileen complained of having a stiff neck, I ran right over and began rubbing her neck and shoulders. Without telling her, I also took the opportunity to use my thoughts and intention to send healing to Eileen through my hands. Within a few minutes, Eileen remarked that her stiff neck was gone. So, of course, Carol had to have a massage, too. "Me next," she said, noting that she had a terrible headache. I obliged, began to rub Carol's temples and head, while also quietly using my thoughts to send healing to her through my hands. Within minutes, Carol's headache had vanished. That was the good news. The bad news was that, also within minutes, I was suffering with a stiff neck and a headache.

So that night, I went home and I thought, "There is something not right here. I cannot help people if I'm going to take on their symptoms and illnesses." So I prayed about this and tried to tune in to my intuition. I had a heart-to-heart talk with God, during which I experienced a strong feeling that I needed to be more grounded and protected. I began tailoring the tools and techniques Holly had taught me, in a way I thought would best support what would soon become my healing work. I began surrounding myself in a bubble of God's white light and imagining that my feet were connected to the center of the earth, like the roots of a big tree (stay tuned for chapter 5). This approach seemed to work: I was able to provide healing to the recipient while protecting myself from taking on his or her symptoms. Miraculously, when I began to apply this method in providing healing to others, I, too, experienced a complete healing from the arthritic pain as well as other ailments I had been experiencing over the past years. I began to understand that I was serving as a channel for God's energy to protect, ground, balance, and ultimately heal the person in spirit, mind, heart, and/or physical body.

As I began working as a healer, I continued to learn about spirituality, energy, balance, wellness, dis-ease, and healing. I learned that it's important to care for our whole selves—all the parts of us. When we don't take care of our spiritual needs, we can become out of balance and this can contribute to symptoms in our spiritual, mental, emotional, and even physical selves. In addition to excellent medical and psychosocial care, each of us is in need of spiritual protection, healing, and care.

Initially, I offered this spiritual care by using my hands, placed on or near the recipient, to provide an energy healing to my clients—men, women, and children who had been diagnosed with or had been experiencing all types of issues, symptoms, and dis-ease. I didn't ask people for feedback, but often was told in session or later that the healing had helped to reduce or eliminate their dis-ease or symptoms. As I continued to see more clients, I also continued to gain knowledge from this experience and to fine-tune my healing approach and techniques. Along the way, I began to see that some people would experience a healing or relief of their symptoms after an energy healing, but over a period of time, may find that the symptoms began to return. I also determined that, contributing to the cause of many of our symptoms and dis-ease are deep hurts and traumas from the past. As in my mother's case, I found that if I could help people identify and resolve these underlying deep hurts that they could induce and maintain a more effective, sustained healing. Through this experience, I learned that healing is not a one-way street. The recipient needs to participate in his or her own healing, initially and on an ongoing basis, in order to correct the underlying causes of the dis-ease and maintain a state of health and balance over time. As a result, I altered my healing sessions to include not only an energy healing, but also a discussion of past hurts and a teaching session on the application of simple "homework" exercises to help people spiritually protect, connect, ground, and maintain balance and healing for themselves. Using this approach, I was blessed to be able to help facilitate the healing process for people with all kinds of symptoms and dis-ease.

When I looked back on my journey, I realized that I am and always have been an empath. As you will soon see, my experiences with illness as a child, the autoimmune and other dis-ease, the sensitivity to medications and fragrances, even my feeling the physical pain of others as my own—these are all traits of an empath. Since I learned to protect, ground, and care for my spiritual self and discover my own spiritual gift, my symptoms have largely disappeared or greatly lessened (although I am still sensitive to fragrances, they no longer send me into anaphylaxis). And while I have never had the symptom of anxiety that I see in so many of my clients who are empaths, I would soon find that, with a little tweaking and innovation, the same approach to spiritual care and healing that helped me could also help them.

So what do you say...shall we find out whether you or your loved one who is suffering with unexplained chronic anxiety or related symptoms just might be an empath?

Pop Quiz Anyone?

As the name suggests, empaths are individuals who possess tremendous empathy for others. Most people have empathy and have empathic traits, but if we think of these traits on a spectrum, I believe empaths would be on the extreme end of that continuum. We may even say they have a kind of turbo-charged empathy. They feel other people's energies, thoughts, and emotions. They feel others' joy and happiness. They feel other people's pain and struggles. They are likely to be highly uncomfortable in situations of discord or disharmony. Empaths often feel the urge to "make better" others' suffering and to play the role of peacemaker in conflict. They may have great concern and compassion for animals and for the earth. While these are beautiful qualities to have, the empaths' highly sensitive nature can result in them feeling overwhelmed by the energies that surround them. I believe this is, in part, because empaths are energy "sponges," not only relating to people's feelings but absorbing these energies—experiencing them as if they are their own, sometimes being unable to tell the difference between their own thoughts, feelings, and energy and those around them. They may even feel or experience these energies, such as physical pain, discomfort, or other symptoms, in their physical bodies.

Could *you* be an empath? Let's start with a quick quiz. Different practitioners or authors may list varying traits of an empath. In the sidebar on page oo, I've listed the traits here that I observe most commonly in my practice. Let's see if any of these resonate for you. Please place a check next to all questions to which you answer yes.

Quiz: Could You Be an Empath?

Check the box for every "yes" answer.

☐ Do you suffer from unexplained anxiety, panic attacks, phobias, or fear?

☐ Do you suffer with unexplained feelings of sadness or depression?

☐ Do people sometimes refer to you as being "sensitive" or "too sensitive"?

☐ Do you suffer with frequent, unexplained headaches?

☐ Do you suffer with unexplained digestive issues, nausea, irritable bowel syndrome, or upset stomach?

☐ Have you been diagnosed with chronic fatigue syndrome, fibromyalgia, or an autoimmune dis-ease?

☐ Do you have difficulty falling asleep or staying asleep?

☐ Do you seem to simply "know" things?

☐ Do you often experience a high-pitched sound or ringing in your ears?

Did you check "yes" to any of the quiz questions? While having one or two of these traits would not be unusual for anyone, if you found yourself responding in the affirmative to several questions, then you could be an empath. As the quiz indicates, the traits of an empath can include not only anxiety and other symptoms, but a range of sensitivities that can span the physical, emotional, and mental domains. In my experience, empaths are individuals who possess a heightened sensitivity to the energy around them. Overall, empaths are highly sensitive people and they may experience this sensitivity in a

☐ Do you seem particularly perceptive about the intentions, motivations, or honesty of others?

☐ Do you have an acute awareness of or take on the feelings or moods of others around you?

☐ Do you feel increased anxiety or discomfort when in a group, crowd, or large social event or setting?

☐ Do you feel others' physical or emotional pain?

☐ Are you especially sensitive to sound, light, or smells?

☐ Are you especially sensitive to medications, chemicals, or fragranced lotions and soaps?

☐ Do you find it unbearable to watch violent or negative television shows, movies, or news coverage?

☐ Do you get sick often or have others referred to you as a hypochondriac?

☐ Do you find that others often come to you with their problems?

☐ Do you feel comforted by sitting with your arms crossed or with a pillow, pet, or other object in front of you?

☐ Do you feel comforted by being in nature?

number of ways. For example, in terms of physical stimuli and reactions, many empaths are especially sensitive to light, sound, and odors. As I've said before, for individuals who have a heightened sensitivity to light, they may have difficulty with bright light, flashing light, or certain types of light. Many empaths I have met, myself included, develop headaches from exposure to fluorescent lights. Others may find themselves squinting when outdoors or may find they need to wear sunglasses more frequently than the average person. Those who are exceptionally sensitive to sound may have a strong reaction or startle reflex to loud noises or to a certain sound type or pitch, or feel overwhelmed by too many noises or too much talking or sound all at once. People who are sensitive to odors may have difficulty with certain types of smells or with strong fragrances such as cigarette smoke or those found in some soaps, detergents, lotions, or candles. They may simply find it unpleasant or may develop symptoms such as headaches when exposed to these smells. Some empaths also seem to be especially sensitive to certain chemicals (such as cleaning products) and medications, and can be susceptible to developing frequent physical illnesses. For this reason, they are sometimes referred to as hypochondriacs by others. This may be due to their developing illnesses as well as to their tendency to feel and take on others' pain and other symptoms as their own.

Beyond these physical sensitivities, we also see that empaths are often highly perceptive about others' thoughts, intentions, and motivations. They seem to just know things. As we noted, empaths have extreme empathy and compassion for others' feelings and situations. They may also find it difficult to watch negatively charged news coverage, violent television programs, or even very sad shows or advertisements. Because they are good listeners and always want to help, they may find that their phones and doorbells are ringing continuously. Many empaths also may have uncomfortable feelings relating to world events or natural disasters. For example, I have students who will experience dreams, visions, messages, or a feeling of somberness or foreboding right before a large-scale flood, earthquake, wildfire, shooting, plane crash, or other situation. They may feel this way before it happens or right as it's happening. After the event transpires, or these individuals become aware that it has transpired, they stop sensing this energy. They are like satellite dishes, picking up information, emotions, and other energy from the Universe all around them.

But what is it that makes an empath so sensitive and susceptible to external energies—whether mental, emotional, or physical? How can they feel or know or otherwise perceive things that are, really if you think about it, beyond the ability of our five physical senses? I believe part of the answer lies in the highly spiritual, intuitive nature of an empath. Indeed, I have found that many empaths possess a heightened sense of intuition and related spiritual gifts.

Heightened Intuition

Understanding the empath starts with understanding that we are all spirit, all made of energy. Each of us is a spiritual being who has been given the privilege of experiencing this wonderful and temporary state of being human. As souls who are undergoing the human experience, we all have spiritual, mental, emotional, and physical selves to tend to and keep in balance. And we are all perceiving, receiving, and transmitting energy, to and from each other and the Universe around us.

As spiritual beings, we all have the gift of intuition. Merriam-Webster defines the word *intuition* as "quick and ready insight; immediate apprehension or cognition; knowledge or conviction gained by intuition; the power or faculty of attaining direct knowledge or cognition without evident rational thought and inference." I would go further and say that intuition is derived from our spiritual nature. I believe our intuition is a fundamental spiritual gift, a sensing, knowing, feeling, or otherwise perceiving that is derived not through our human experience or the normal range of our five physical senses, but through our connection to our own spiritual selves and to God and the Universe around us. Some would call this extrasensory perception.

Our gift of intuition is ours to help guide us for the entire length of our days here on earth (and beyond). We often experience our intuition as that still small voice, or that inner feeling, inside of us. If we listen, if we pay attention, we can hear that still small voice or feel our own inner compass whispering to us, guiding us, protecting and in some cases warning us, and ultimately pushing us forward to the light of our own destinies. We can use our powers of intuition to perceive energy and discern information from external sources, like other people, animals, places, and spaces. In many cases, when we experience this energy, it can manifest as a strong *sense* of *feeling*. I believe this sense of *feeling* is often perceived and absorbed through our solar plexus chakra, which I sometimes refer to as the *seat of intuition*. The solar plexus chakra is one of the body's main *chakras*—or wheels or centers of energy— and is located between the navel and breastbone. Indeed, some may say it is right over the gut. Over time, I have also come to believe that some people may also perceive or absorb the sense of feeling through the heart chakra, located in the area of the chest. Have you ever had or heard of a "gut feeling," "gut instinct," or "butterflies in the stomach"? Or have you ever felt someone watching you, had the hair on the back of your neck stand up, or felt goose bumps up and down your arms? That's your intuition.

For people who are *empaths*, I believe this sense of intuition is heightened and contributing to the individuals' exceptional perception of and sensitivity to the external energies around them. As we noted, an empath perceives, takes in, and I believe absorbs and holds on to the energy, feelings, moods, thoughts, and intentions of other people, animals, places, and spaces.

While our intuition may be sensed in one or more of several different ways, I have found that this enhanced state of perception for empaths who suffer with anxiety tends to include a strong sense of feeling. For example, an empath may visit a museum and experience the energy from hundreds of ancient art pieces and artifacts—some good, some not so good. She may walk into a large group at school, work, or a social event and feel the thoughts and emotions of every person around her. In many cases, empaths may experience these energies as their own—thoughts, intentions, and emotions from happy to depressed to angry to worried and fearful—and not realize that it's *not* coming from themselves. Many empaths will not realize why they are feeling this way, and will simply develop an aversion to or fear of groups or public places. This alone can be overwhelming for empaths, causing them to feel drained, exhausted, and yes, anxious.

But now, consider this: In my experience, our intuition can allow us to connect with and perceive energies not only from human beings, animals, places, and objects—but also those from the spirit world. This means that when an empath walks into that social event, he may not only feel the energies of the human beings who are there, but perhaps also the significant number of beings in spirit form who are with those people! Without preventive measures in place, this can happen to empaths whether or not they want it to and whether or not they realize it.

Over the years, I have found that when empathic individuals do not understand that they are perceiving, sensing, and experiencing the external energies around them (whether from this world or the spirit world), and do not have the simple tools to protect their energy in this state of heightened sensitivity, they can develop one or more of a constellation of symptoms. You guessed it: anxiety, anxiety, and more anxiety—as well as chronic panic attacks, phobias, feelings of sadness or depression, nausea, digestive issues, chronic fatigue, frequent headaches, and other dis-ease. This type of anxiety, along with other symptoms, is not coming from simply being nervous about attending an event. It's coming from the empath's feeling and absorbing external energies into his or her own chakras and energy field.

Just as our intuition enables us to sense the energies around us, our intuition also can allow us to connect and communicate directly with our own higher spiritual selves, our spirit guides, our loved ones who are in spirit form, and with God. And just like our intuition in other areas, our perception of energy from the spirit world can come to us in many different ways. Each and every one of us possesses this beautiful gift of connection with the spiritual realm. I believe that our intuition can manifest as, or be the facilitator for, more specific spiritual gifts such as the ability to receive or discern information from the Universe and energy around us (often referred to as intuitive or psychic ability), ability to communicate directly with beings in the spirit world (often referred to as mediumship or psychic mediumship), spiritual healing, and others. I believe we may all have these spiritual gifts to some degree, but because empaths have a heightened sense of underlying intuition, they may also possess one or more exceptionally strong spiritual gifts such as these.

For those who have strong underlying psychic or mediumship gifts, their abilities can manifest as feeling, seeing, hearing, tasting, smelling, or simply knowing the presence of spiritual beings, energy, or information. This does not mean that most people see spirits standing in front of them or hear someone else's voice speaking to them. Although some people do experience this, for most individuals I have met, the perception or "communication" comes less dramatically. For example, they may see an image of someone or something (like a place, a word, a thing) in their mind or mind's eye, or hear a message that comes in their own inner voice. They may catch a glimpse of something out of the corner of their eye, but when they look, it's gone. They may feel someone sit on their bed at night, only to find that no one is there. They may smell their late grandfather's cigar smoke. They may receive messages during vivid dreams or may be unable to sleep or be awakened frequently due to spiritual "visitors" in the night. These types of experiences often go unnoticed. However, if these intuitive gifts are recognized and developed, they may yield the capability of more sustained, controlled connection and communication with the spirit world and the Universe around us. . In the case of those with strong spiritual healing gifts, many are able to see, feel, or know about another person's dis-ease or even feel their emotional or physical pain. Often, this is accompanied by the urge to make it better and, in some cases, having extra warm or hot hands.

I believe some of the symptoms or traits attributed to being an empath are due directly to the extreme spiritual gifts that so many empaths possess but do not know they have. I find that most people with these gifts are completely unaware of them, dismiss them as imagination or intrusive or random thoughts, or are afraid of them and deliberately hide or suppress them. I have observed that, especially for those like myself with strong healing abilities, their heightened state of sensitivity without the needed awareness and care, over time, can contribute to frequent illnesses and the development of conditions such as chronic fatigue, digestive symptoms, autoimmune, and other dis-ease. Indeed, in my experience (so far) many whose gifts manifest primarily as healing abilities tend to present with these types of conditions, and less commonly with anxiety. But for those who turn out to have exceptional (although undiscovered) psychic and mediumship abilities, I have found that chronic anxiety (along with digestive issues, frequent headaches, and numerous other symptoms) is a particularly common symptom. In fact, the majority of people who have come to me suffering with unexplained chronic anxiety have been empaths who also had exceptionally strong hidden psychic or mediumship abilities. This does not mean that they are meant to become professional psychics or mediums necessarily, or even that they are all meant to provide intuitive messages or "readings" to others. For many, it simply means that they possess and can discover and develop their gifts so that they can use them to guide and enhance their own lives. Ultimately opening to their whole selves, including their spiritual gifts, helps them to be the best parents, friends, doctors, nurses, police officers, firefighters, artists, teachers, and human beings they can be.

It is important to note that, while our gift of intuition is with us always, there are times in our lives when we may experience an especially heightened sense of intuition and sense of spirituality. This often happens when we are transitioning from one developmental stage of our lives to another or when we are experiencing significant hormonal fluctuations or other changes. We have all heard of a "mid-life crisis." And we know that our teenage years can be challenging, as we move from childhood into adulthood. I believe these are times not only of emotional, mental, and other developmental growth, but also of increased spirituality and spiritual growth. They are phases during which we are often searching for deeper connection, meaning, and truth in our lives. As such, these can also be especially vulnerable periods. This is true for all of us, but for an empath who experiences a heightened sense of intuition already, the effect of these periods can be even more dramatic, with an emergence, re-emergence, or escalation of symptoms. Being aware of these especially sensitive or vulnerable phases of life can help us to identify ourselves, children, or other loved ones as potential empaths and, when needed, to take extra measures to protect, ground, and balance.

INFANCY. In infancy, we enter into our earthly lives and are still very much connected to the spirit world. All babies may have a heightened sense of intuition. However, if a baby is an empath, you may notice that she is perfectly comfortable and peaceful in her own home or with her core family, but becomes inconsolable or has difficulty eating or sleeping when in a crowd or more social setting.

TODDLER AGE. Toddlers are still highly open to their spiritual selves and, as we know, sometimes develop imaginary friends. As a spiritual healer and teacher, I have to say that sometimes these playmates are imaginary and sometimes not. A toddler who is an empath with strong spiritual gifts may look at things or talk to people whom others do not see or hear, draw pictures of places they have never been, or talk about things they have no earthly way of knowing. I cannot provide a medical assessment, but from a spiritual perspective, I find all of this to be absolutely fine unless it becomes troublesome or frightening to the child. They may show a fear of being alone (especially at night), but in my experience, this usually starts when they are a little older. As with infants, toddlers who are empaths also may cry or develop anxiety or social withdrawal in crowds or social gatherings.

SCHOOL AGE. When children enter elementary school, they begin to exercise more use of the left brain and their spiritual connection can become less overt or pronounced. However, this does not mean they stop being spiritual beings. While many children can experience some stress around entering into the school setting, this can be exacerbated in those who are empaths. Children who are empaths can experience anxiety, panic, phobias, feelings of sadness or depression, upset stomach, headaches, and sometimes attention issues when they enter school and begin feeling and absorbing the energies of the new people and places in their lives. Those who experience strong spiritual gifts may demonstrate similar behaviors as toddlers—such as speaking or writing with a knowledge that is beyond their own life experience and hearing from or seeing people or "faces" who are in spirit form. At this age, they are also more likely than younger children to display fear of these experiences—such as being afraid of going to bed at night, being afraid of the dark or of being left alone, and experiencing night terrors. They may begin to hide these experiences and fears, if they can, as they begin to realize that this is not the socially accepted "norm."

PUBERTY. At the time of puberty, hormones are changing and children can again experience a rise in their spirituality and heightened sensitivities. For adolescents who are empaths or who have spiritual gifts of which they are unaware or afraid, anxiety, panic attacks, phobias, feelings of sadness or depression, frequent headaches, and related symptoms may develop. This may manifest in a number of ways, including withdrawal from social activities, self-medication with drugs and alcohol, cutting, or other self-destructive activities. Again, this can be true for all teenagers who are making their way through this challenging age, but it can be especially pronounced in empaths.

ADULTHOOD. Other periods of increased spiritual sensitivity may occur during times of pregnancy, the postpartum period, menopause, or what we often refer to as a mid-life crisis for both men and women. Changing hormones can make us more sensitive to all energy and sensory perceptions, including those that are spiritual. Often, a "mid-life crisis" is merely a longing for a deeper and more meaningful connection to our spiritual selves. This is true for all individuals, but can be exacerbated in empathic individuals, who may also experience a re-emergence or intensification of anxiety, panic, phobias, depression, or other symptoms, or of any unrealized or suppressed spiritual gifts during these phases of life. Strong spiritual gifts can become even more heightened or overt during these times.

While these time periods represent those of potentially increased sensitivity for empaths (and indeed, for everyone), an empath's heightened sense of intuition is also part of his or her life each and every day—and related symptoms can occur at any time. Increased vigilance is needed during these transition phases, but as we will soon see (chapters 5–8), the use of our spiritual connection and thought exercises to protect, ground, and balance is needed on an ongoing, daily basis. Depending on age, individuals can perform the needed exercises themselves or can be assisted, in an age-appropriate way, by an adult.

Ultimately, while empaths can be highly sensitive and susceptible to many types of energies—spiritual (beings in spirit form, spiritual energy), mental (thoughts, intentions, motivations), emotional (moods, feelings), and physical (such as light, sounds, fragrances, chemicals, foods)—I often refer to the symptoms they develop as "spiritually based."

This is because I believe the root of many of these symptoms is, at least in part, the empath's heightened sense of intuition, which is of a spiritual nature or the nature of their spiritual being on earth.

Could This Be You?

For so many of my clients and students who were empaths, the energies they had been experiencing and absorbing, without the awareness and protection they needed, were overwhelming and led to what I consider spiritually based suffering. However, once these beautiful, sensitive people realized they were empaths (and many of them, also with strong hidden psychic and mediumship abilities), they were able to take some simple steps to protect themselves, eliminate or significantly reduce their anxiety, and begin to open to their whole selves and live the lives for which they were destined. While I did not know the life stories or backgrounds of most of my clients and students when I first saw them, some of them have graciously agreed to share their stories here, so that others who are struggling with spiritually based anxiety or other empath-related symptoms may find their way to health and wholeness.

Nick

Several years ago, Nick received a reading with spiritual medium Diana Cinquemani, who happened to be one of my students, for his seventeenth birthday. When Diana heard about the anxiety with which he had been suffering, she recommended that he see me.

Nick began attending my spiritual awareness classes, and one night approached me after class and told me about the severe anxiety and panic attacks he had been experiencing for as long as he could remember. At night, he was so anxious that he couldn't sleep and didn't want to be alone in his room. He had never tried medication for his anxiety, but he had seen a therapist when he was in middle school. He had found his therapist to be tremendously helpful in discussing his issues and feelings, but his anxiety remained unchanged.

I felt so badly for this young man when he told me that his anxiety had intensified when he reached high school and now was at the point that he was having difficulty functioning in a public setting. He continued going to school, but he could no longer participate in sports and he had isolated himself socially. His anxiety had become debilitating, and as a result, he was also feeling depressed. I explained to Nick that he is an empath and needs to protect himself spiritually. Initially, I gave him three key tools—my surround, ground, and shield exercises, all done by thought—to apply every day to protect and balance his energy, shield his solar plexus and heart from negative and toxic energies, and alleviate his anxiety.

Nick could not believe how quickly these tools worked for him. He said he felt in control of his life again and no longer felt at the mercy of the energies and emotions around him. Like so many empaths, Nick also turned out to be a talented spiritual medium. For this reason, I also asked Nick to post, just using his thoughts, a spiritual Do Not Disturb sign to let those in spirit form know that he did not wish to communicate at certain times of the day and night (such as when he was supposed to be sleeping).

As of this writing, Nick has graduated from nursing school and is working in a hospital. I am happy to say that he also has a social life. Nick says he's come full circle, having started out needing all the help he could get and now feeling blessed to be able to use his gifts to help others.

Candace

Candace was a wife and stay-at-home mother of two who thought she was in perfect health when, one day, she was making breakfast and passed out without warning. She told me that she was subsequently diagnosed with autonomic dysfunction, a condition in which the autonomic nervous system is damaged or is not functioning properly. In Candace's case, this resulted in her heartbeat being difficult to control, her blood pressure becoming dangerously high or low, and sudden fainting spells. Candace's condition ultimately worsened to the point that she could not drive, had to be careful on stairs, and had difficulty digesting food. She developed chronic fatigue and became so sick that her husband would have to carry her upstairs to bed every night. Unfortunately, her doctor indicated that there was no medication, surgery, or other therapy that could help her. In addition to this medical condition, Candace also suffered with anxiety in crowded areas.

Candace learned about my healing work after reading Theresa Caputo's book *There's More to Life Than This*, and hoped that I could help her. When she came to see me in 2013, I talked with her, did an energy healing, and gave her all of my homework exercises—including surround, ground, and shield—to shield her solar plexus and heart from negative or toxic energy, balance and align her energy, and help with her symptoms. Candace, who is an empath, says that she felt better immediately after her session. While she still has autonomic dysfunction, her symptoms have lessened, she has not passed out again, and her husband no longer has to carry her up the stairs to bed. So too, her anxiety is gone and she no longer needs to avoid being in groups or crowds. She jokes that, while her husband doesn't believe in "this stuff," even he admits that it's changed her life. Candace also has the spiritual gifts of both mediumship and healing and is now embracing this part of herself.

Kristianne

Kristianne says that she had suffered with anxiety her whole life. When she was young, she would see and hear people and things that others did not see and hear. She prayed to stop seeing and hearing these things, and she did. But she then developed anxiety and attention deficit disorder (ADD). When she went into crowds or groups, her stomach would be in knots. Her heart would race. At night, she couldn't sleep. In high school and college, she went to doctors and was diagnosed with generalized anxiety disorder, but her symptoms persisted.

When I saw Kristianne in the fall of 2014, I told her what I have told so many others. She is an empath and, in her case, she might also have strong spiritual gifts, all of which can contribute to anxiety and sleeplessness. I gave Kristianne several new tools to protect and balance herself and set boundaries for the energies around her. I instructed her in how to use her thoughts to surround, ground, and shield. As with Nick, I explained to Kristianne that, using her thoughts, she needed to hang a spiritual Do Not Disturb sign at bedtime so she would not be inundated with energies while she was trying to sleep. Using these simple techniques, Kristianne was able to manage her anxiety and begin sleeping through the night for the first time in her life.

Kristianne went on to receive her master's degree and is now a school counselor for elementary and middle school students. She continues to develop her own spiritual gifts and wants to let others know that they don't have to live in fear and anxiety. Reach out, she says, because when you do it's the first day of the rest of your life.

Jen

Jen had been a teacher for fourteen years. She says she loved her work, teaching health class to fifteen- and sixteen-year-olds, but she was suffering with anxiety. She didn't understand why she had the anxiety: She had a good and happy life. She noticed that her symptoms had increased after her grandfather died ten years before and that they were exacerbated in groups, including with the students she loved so much. The anxiety would subside a bit in the summer, and then regain intensity when school would begin in the fall. She had tried meditation—and even taught "meditation Mondays" to her students—and found this very helpful. But still her anxiety persisted. She would find herself talking a mile a minute, getting worked up about something she felt she needed to get out. Yet, she didn't know what it was or why she was feeling this way. It just didn't make sense to her.

One day, she complimented one of her students on her miraculous medal, a gift given to her by her grandmother. That student happened to be my granddaughter, and in October 2015, Jen came to me for a healing session for her anxiety. In this case, the teacher went home with the homework. I asked Jen to use her thoughts to surround, ground, and shield every single day. I also gave her my Universal White Light Meditation, to help her to spiritually connect, ground, and balance. Jen says she experienced a reduction in her anxiety and felt lighter, grateful, and more hopeful "pretty much immediately." She continues to teach meditation to her students, stressing the importance of using positive thought, focusing on strengths, and practicing gratitude. She encourages others to listen to their own inner guidance, telling them that it doesn't come as a lightning bolt, but in your own voice, in a whisper.

Jessica

Jessica was married at twenty years old. When her marriage ended, she developed debilitating anxiety. She experienced anxiety every single day, she had insomnia, and began having difficulty interacting with people, both one-on-one and in groups. Ultimately, she obtained a job that allowed her to work from home and avoid going out. Jessica tried antianxiety and antidepressant medications, acupuncture, and herbal therapies. She said these interventions would work for a few hours and then her anxiety would return.

In December 2015, she and her sister attended one of my seminars on "Bridging the Gap Between Anxiety and Mediumship." During the seminar, I gave a quiz to see how many attendees had the traits of an empath and then did a healing meditation. Jessica answered yes to multiple quiz questions, and during the meditation found herself relaxing, taking off her jacket, uncrossing her arms, and looking around to connect with other people. After the meditation, I instructed attendees in the surround, ground, and shield exercises, so that they could go home with the tools they needed to protect and balance themselves in their day-to-day lives.

Jessica uses these tools every day. She says she has no anxiety whatsoever, is able to sleep through the night, and has begun to accept her own spiritual gifts.

Jennifer

I was speaking at an event recently, when a woman walked up and gave me the biggest hug as she cried and thanked me for helping her sister, Jennifer. Standing next to her was Jennifer, a client who had also become a student of mine. Jennifer was a forty-three-year-old wife and mother of two who had experienced debilitating depression all of her life. She had told me that she had attempted suicide three times, the first time at only four years old.

Jennifer would hear constant chatter in her head and would see things that other people didn't see. Unable to understand where these intrusive visions and sounds were coming from, she would become very depressed. Her doctors did their best to help her. Jennifer reported that she had tried multiple medications, including anti-depressants, antipsychotics, and antianxiety agents. Over the course of her life, Jennifer says she had been in and out of psychiatric hospitals several times and had undergone twenty-four rounds of bilateral electroshock therapy to the brain. But the chatter and seeing things would always start up again, and she would go into another deep depression. She wondered how she could go on like this.

Then, out of the blue, a friend asked Jennifer if she had seen the *Long Island Medium* on television. She checked it out, loved Theresa and loved the show, and somehow found her way to my website. At that time, Jennifer had been experiencing anxiety along with severe depression. She says she had just been discharged from the hospital, had tried everything else, and thought "what the heck, why not try this."

In January 2016, Jennifer, who has an angelic presence, came to see me for a healing session. I talked with her, told her she is an empath, did an energy healing, and gave her all the homework, including the surround, ground, and shield exercises and Universal White Light Meditation. Since that time, Jennifer has started attending my monthly spiritual awareness class and working to develop her spiritual gifts. You see, Jennifer has been a spiritual medium her whole life and had stuffed all that energy down. Now she has been able to control and make friends with the chatter in her head and it has brought what she calls "an amazing peace and a hope" that she has never had before. Not surprisingly, Jennifer is also blessed with the gift of spiritual healing. Over time, she has worked with her physician to taper down the dosage of her medications, and she eventually was able to discontinue them. Her whole life, Jennifer wanted to die. Today, she is embracing her gifts of spiritual healing and mediumship and is grateful to be able to share them with others in need. Today, Jennifer wants to live.

I am forever grateful to these brave and gifted souls and to so many others for sharing their stories, so that others who are struggling may be able to learn from them, see themselves in their experiences, and find their way to healing and wholeness. All of these individuals are empaths who presented with anxiety or other empath-related symptoms that I believe were being caused, at least in part, by factors of a spiritual nature. I believe it is important for people to see their physicians, therapists, and other health professionals for anxiety, panic attacks, depression, or any physical or mental symptoms or conditions they may have. At the same time, it's also important to take care of our spiritual selves—and medication is not always the answer or the complete answer. All of these individuals, some of whom had suffered with their conditions for years, were able to reduce their symptoms significantly by applying a few simple exercises—all done by thought—to protect, ground, and balance themselves in spirit-mind-heart-body.

Could this be you? If you answered yes to several quiz questions, or if you saw yourself in the stories of Nick, Candace,

Kristianne, Jen, Jessica, or Jennifer, then it's possible that you too could be an empath. Let's learn a little more about the connection between anxiety and spirit, and how I came to discover that some very simple tools can help eliminate this type of anxiety and related symptoms.

CHAPTER 2

Making the Connection
between Anxiety and Spirit

I N THE BEGINNING OF MY work as a spiritual healer, I
found that I tended to meet clusters of people, often in
threes, who shared the same symptoms or conditions. It was
as though the Universe was bringing us together, both to help
the clients and to teach me about the different manifestations
and phases of illness. Ultimately, I began to see countless num-
bers of people having been diagnosed with all types of
"dis-ease," from digestive issues to autoimmune dis-ease to
neurologic conditions to cancer. Before long, I also found myself seeing anxiety, anxiety, and more anxiety, both in my
healing practice and in my spiritual awareness class.

I am not referring to the experience of occasional or temporary bouts of anxiety, which most people might feel when
they are nervous or concerned about something like an upcoming test, medical report, job interview, or even a first date.
The people I was seeing were reporting chronic, persistent, se-

35

vere, sometimes debilitating anxiety. And the anxiety did not come alone. People would come in desperate with panic attacks, irrational fears, feelings of sadness or depression, frequent headaches, and a whole constellation of symptoms. Many would describe lifelong anxiety, while others would note symptoms that began after certain events or losses in their lives. They would report feeling overly or persistently jittery, restless, worried, concerned, or fearful; having sudden feelings of panic or "fight or flight response"; developing phobias like a fear or aversion to driving; being in a crowd, having to interact with people, or leaving the confines of their home; having difficulty sleeping and physical symptoms of feeling their heart racing or pounding or their stomach in knots. Some would experience frequent headaches or intense bouts of nausea and digestive issues. Others said they had suffered with feelings of sadness or depression along with their anxiety, sometimes since childhood, and they just didn't know why. Often they would come after seeing physicians and therapists and trying medications and other interventions, with little or no relief. While I found I was able to help many people with a healing session or with spiritual awareness lessons, it wasn't until my experience with a certain Long Island Medium that I began to make the full connection between our spiritual traits and the development of anxiety and other symptoms.

I had known Theresa Caputo all of her life. Her mother and I were friends. Theresa and her brother had gone to school with my children. I had seen her friendly, bubbly self at school events, sports activities, house parties, you name it. Yet I had not been aware of the terrible anxiety that had plagued her for years. Little did I know that, as a child, she had suffered from night terrors. She had been afraid to be alone at night. As she entered into her adolescence and adulthood, she noticed more and more that she would experience anxiety or just didn't feel right around different people and places. After she had her two children, whom she loved dearly, her anxiety had intensified. By the time she entered into her late twenties, her anxiety was off the charts and she was suffering with a host of phobias.

It was a number of years after I had begun practicing as a healer and teacher that Theresa's mother had invited me to her home to attend a scented-candle party, which was kind of a thing back then. I happily accepted the invitation (despite my sensitivity to the fragrances), and it was there, at this candle party of all places, that I first noticed that Theresa seemed to be having some anxiety among the crowd. Then out of nowhere, from across the room I heard that voice, "Mrs. Longo, are you a psychic?" I explained to Theresa that I was a spiritual healer, and she asked if I could do a healing for her. It was the end of the party, and Theresa and I were able to find a quiet room where we could be alone. I asked to be a channel by which God could provide His light and healing energy for the highest good of all concerned, and I placed my hands over Theresa's head and began an overall healing, sometimes called an "energy healing." Since I had noticed earlier that Theresa seemed to have some anxiety, I also focused on giving her healing for this issue specifically.

I still did not realize the extent of Theresa's struggle with anxiety, not until she called a few weeks following the party. Theresa said she had felt calmer than she had in years. Her husband Larry had noticed this and suggested that she may want to schedule another healing. I told her she didn't need another session at that time if she was feeling well.

Later, I would learn more about the anxiety, panic attacks, and phobias with which Theresa had been struggling. Her symptoms had escalated over time, and she had been having difficulty with driving, riding in a car, taking an elevator, flying in an airplane, being in a group of people, and other ordinary, everyday activities that many of us take for granted. Her fear had been paralyzing, and she had been seeing a therapist to try to resolve it. She said her therapist had told her she had "anticipatory anxiety"—but she didn't know why she was experiencing this. Theresa had had a happy upbringing and had a beautiful family, with a supportive husband and parents. Yet her anxiety had persisted.

Ultimately, the spiritual healing session had helped to restore balance and alleviate Theresa's anxiety—but initially I didn't have an understanding of what had caused her symptoms in the first place. At this point in my work, I understood the importance of spiritual connection, protection, grounding, and balance. I knew that we all have a still small voice or feeling inside, or sense of intuition, that guides us on our earthly journey. I knew that some people, called empaths, possess a heightened sense of intuition, including a high sensitivity to the energy around them, and often perceive, feel, and absorb the energy of other people, places, and things. I also knew that, for many of these individuals, this heightened sense of intuition could also manifest as exceptionally strong spiritual gifts. I was also starting to put together that many of my clients and students who had a strong ability to communicate with the spirit world seemed to experience anxiety as well. But it just hadn't quite clicked. I still didn't fully understand that this heightened sense of perception or sensitivity and these exceptional spiritual gifts and abilities, if not recognized, cared for, and embraced, could result in the perfect storm of anxiety, panic, irrational fears, phobias, frequent headaches, and other symptoms. And while our initial spiritual healing session had helped, over time, Theresa's anxiety would begin to reemerge.

When Theresa eventually began attending my spiritual awareness class in 2002 or so, she proved to be an incredibly quick and diligent student. As it turned out, Theresa had an extremely heightened sense of intuition. She was, in fact, an empath and a gifted spiritual medium, meaning she could communicate with and receive messages from beings in the spirit world. Who knew? Not me. Not her. But one of the other mediums in class, who was also highly gifted, had recognized Theresa's hidden abilities early on. In the very first week, she had commented to Theresa that this was going to go very fast for her. To this Theresa had replied something like, "This what, what is this?" By the second week of class, Theresa was speaking to people's loved ones in the spirit world and delivering clear and accurate messages to classmates and guests. Let me tell you, this freaked her out. I can still hear her, insisting that she wasn't the one getting these messages, that it was only happening because she was sitting in another medium's chair that day. She thought it must have rubbed off on her, but it was sure to go away. But Theresa's gifts would no longer be denied, and her progress was rapid.

At that time, I would often schedule readings for the advanced students in class so they could begin to share their gifts and further develop their skills. At one point, we were offered an opportunity to give readings to the clients at a nearby hair salon, and I invited Theresa to join us. This would be her first session for real clients and I was excited for her. There was only one problem. Theresa did not want to go. She argued, she debated, she said she wasn't ready. She was terrified. However, in the end, she did go and she was able to provide readings for several salon clients that day. She did incredibly well, and she was able to see the healing effects that her gift could bring to those in need. Afterward, Theresa told me something I will never forget. As soon as we walked out of the building, she grabbed my arm, looked at me with tears in her eyes and said, "I feel whole for the first time in my life."

This is when it all began to click for me. I found this moment to be profoundly moving, and it became one that would compel a shift in my understanding about the nature of the anxiety and other symptoms I had been seeing in many of my clients and students. I began to realize that Theresa had had this gift all of her life. She had been able to see, hear, and feel beings in spirit form and their energy since she was four years old, but did not understand this. She didn't know what it was or what to do with it, so she tried to ignore or dismiss it. With this, the messages, which come through energy, kept coming. And when the energy was pushed away or pushed down, like a giant beach ball being submerged under the ocean, it just kept pushing its way back up to the surface. I believe it was this lack of awareness and suppression of her gift, the denial of her whole self, that had caused this powerful spiritual energy to come bubbling up as extreme anxiety, panic, and phobias. I also believe that, the way Theresa would receive some of her messages also contributed to her anxiety and phobias. While mediums can receive their messages in a number of ways (visit chapter 9), one of the ways that Theresa receives messages is in a sense of *feeling* what our loved ones in spirit form are conveying. For example, Theresa may experience difficulty breathing or discomfort in the chest area when communicating with someone who died of pneumonia. This would cause anxiety and panic in almost anyone, unless they know why it's happening and how to stop it.

In coming to class and using the Universal White Light Meditation (chapter 5), Theresa was able to continue to ground and balance herself and to further develop and utilize her spiritual gift of mediumship to help others. With this, the anxiety, panic, phobias, and fear that had been her lifelong companions began to subside. I was amazed by this—and I had to wonder whether this same phenomenon could be an underlying cause of the anxiety and related symptoms I had been seeing in other clients and students. Had they all been empaths in need of better tools to protect their energy? Were they being inundated by the energies around them, including those from the spirit world? Had they, like Theresa, spent their entire lives never knowing what it is to feel whole?

Indeed, as I continued to work with others who came to me with anxiety, I observed over and over again that, like Theresa, many were empaths. Unaware of this, they were living, in essence, spiritually wide open and unprotected from outside energies. Also like Theresa, almost all were either unaware of or otherwise knowingly or unknowingly dismissing or suppressing their intuitive gifts. They did not *know* their whole selves, let alone love and honor their whole selves. They were fighting their own truth, their own soul's destiny, and it was making them sick. And that's when I knew: Many individuals who are empaths, have strong unrealized or suppressed spiritual gifts (especially those related to psychic or mediumship abilities), or both can be especially susceptible to developing anxiety and related symptoms. I also knew that these symptoms could be alleviated and prevented through spiritual awareness, protection, and care.

In the years following the day Theresa told me that she felt "whole for the first time," I was blessed to be able to help facilitate and teach spiritual healing and care for countless adults and children struggling with all kinds of dis-ease, including anxiety and related symptoms. I continued to offer healing sessions, seminars, webinars, and classes—and I thought I was reaching a lot of people. However, it was only after I appeared with Theresa on the *Long Island Medium* in 2012 that I began to realize just how many others were struggling with chronic, unexplained anxiety. I was inundated with calls, e-mails, and letters from all over the world—many from parents with children who were suffering—hoping that if I could help Theresa, maybe I could help them. After responding to as many people as I could, I became acutely aware that this kind of suffering is much more widespread than I had appreciated and that I could not possibly meet, speak, or Skype individually with every person in need. At that time, it became a priority for me to develop even more simple, more targeted, more easily teachable, and more effective spiritual tools to help empaths—and everyone—to protect and heal themselves from the spiritual causes of their symptoms. I have been grateful to see so many people use these tools to free themselves from their symptoms—and often, quite quickly.

In looking back, I had felt terribly saddened when I realized that Theresa and so many others had suffered for so long with such excruciating symptoms that, in the end, were significantly alleviated with some simple steps. If only I could have figured it out sooner. However, I also came to understand and accept that these challenging experiences are what have allowed us to learn and to grow and have made it possible for so many others to be healed.

Each of us has our own soul's purpose in this lifetime. In Theresa's case, I believe she was chosen to work as a spiritual medium to bring God's message of love, light, and healing to the world. Through her efforts, more people now know that their loved ones who have passed are alive, well, and still with us. So too, Theresa's courage in sharing her story has inspired others who have had similar experiences of anxiety and related symptoms to ask whether they, too, may need spiritual healing or have hidden spiritual gifts to discover and develop. In addition, Theresa and so many others have been teachers to me in my work as a healer, allowing me to better identify, understand, and help individuals who are empaths or have spiritual gifts in need of nurturing.

Through our connection with the Divine, each of us possesses within us the power to care for our spiritual selves; to awaken the power within; and to live our best and most fulfilled lives. We just need the guidance, the *awareness*, to connect with that power. Spiritual healer that I am, I would like to make this information available to everyone. I would like to shout it from the mountaintops! But let me just say it here, for you. If you are struggling with spiritually based anxiety, panic attacks, phobias, or other empath-related symptoms, you don't have to live like this. You don't!

In the chapters ahead, you will find the guidance and simple tools you need to use your thoughts to help heal, care for, and protect yourself spiritually; to discover and begin to develop your own unique gifts of intuition; and to feel whole . . . maybe for the first time in *your* life.

CHAPTER 3

Thoughts Become Things

A T THE BEGINNING OF MY own journey to become more spiritually aware and connected, I started to honor myself, began to tune in to my own inner voice, prayed a lot, and read hundreds of books. I learned a tremendous amount about spirituality and the spiritual self from authors like Echo Bodine, Wayne Dyer, Shakti Gawain, Esther and Jerry Hicks, Florence Scovel Shinn, and many others. One of the most important lessons I learned in my search was something I think I had always known: that we are spiritual beings who are co-creating our own lives through the power of thought. *Thoughts become things.*

I believe that, in addition to our connection with our spiritual selves, this may be the most fundamental universal principle to understand for healing and, well, for living. *Thoughts become things.* Our thoughts become our reality. Every moment of every day we are using our thoughts to manifest our lives. For better or worse, the thoughts we choose to focus on define who we are and who we will be. Think about it. We set our intentions by thought. We dream, aspire, and create by thought. Everything we say and do is preceded by a thought. We can change our mood or feelings by thought. We are the writers, producers, and directors of our own lives—and it all starts with thought. Indeed, our thoughts are an important means by which we are able to connect with our spiritual selves, God, and the Universe around us. Our thoughts can be the difference between fear and faith, between prison and freedom.

When I came to understand this truth fully, I was elated. I wish we all could learn this principle in kindergarten! This means that at any point in time—indeed, at *every* point of time—each of us has within us the power to change our lives, and change the Universe, for the better.

Our thoughts are powerful pulses of energy, being projected into a world that is made of energy. Because we can consciously set our intention and direct our thoughts as we wish, our thoughts can be used to influence our own energy and the energy that exists all around us. Now I am not a physicist. I cannot explain quantum theory to you or give you the mathematical formulas to explain the complexities of the Universe. But in my experience as a spiritual healer, I have come to believe that we are, and everything around us is, made of and hold energy, moving at different vibrations and frequencies. People, animals, insects, trees, air, fire, water, earth, even rocks are made of energy.

As spiritual beings having a human experience, it's as though each of us is our own unique horizon, a meeting of heaven and earth. We are multidimensional beings, possessing what some refer to as the spiritual, mental, emotional, and physical bodies or selves. These four bodies are made of energy, constantly moving at different vibrations and frequencies and thus also having different densities. The energy of our spiritual and mental bodies, for example, is lighter and can be quicker to change than that of our physical bodies. But our physical bodies, too, though they appear solid, are made of energy. While our four bodies hold different energetic vibrations, they still interact, intermingle with, and influence each other.

Further serving to integrate and maintain our flow of energy are *chakras,* often called the body's wheels or centers of energy, where physical matter and consciousness conjoin. We have many chakras, including seven main chakras that align vertically along the spine and head—located at the tailbone, sacrum, solar plexus, heart, throat, third eye (forehead/eyebrow), and crown of the head. Each of the chakras corresponds to a different area of the physical body. Finally, through our chakras and four bodies each of us has flowing through us a Universal spiritual energy or life force (I believe from God), sometimes referred to as "prana" or "chi" or even "breath." All of this energy together—flowing within and through our four bodies and chakras and extending out past the physical body—is sometimes referred to as our energy field, auric field, or aura.

Thought, too, is energy. Indeed, Shakti Gawain called thought a "quick, light, mobile form of energy." This is important because it means that we can change, direct, or redirect our thoughts instantly. In our thoughts, our results can be immediate. The power of an individual thought depends on whether we send it with intention and how much focus or attention we give to it. Our thoughts begin in the mind, or the mental body. If we have a certain thought pop into our mind, but we do not focus on it, it is likely to float or fade away. However, if we focus on or hold on to a certain thought, or send it with intention, the energy of that thought gains power and may expand from the mental body into the emotional body and become an emotion or feeling. If we continue to hold on to that thought and now feeling, it can move into the physical body as well. In some instances, this process can happen almost as quickly as the thought itself. For example, if we are worrying about something, perhaps a speech we have to give, we may quickly experience that thought move into the emotional body, causing anxiety and fear, and into the physical body causing nausea or an upset stomach. On a more positive note, if we find ourselves thinking about a new love in our life, we may quickly experience that thought progressing to feelings of love and joy in our hearts and "butterflies" in our stomachs. In other cases, a thought or feeling can manifest in the physical form—as health or as dis-ease—over years of repetitious thinking in a certain way or about a particular experience or idea.

It's important and empowering to realize the significant impact that our thoughts have on our entire being. It's also important to know that, in addition to having an impact on the state of our own energy, our thoughts can have an effect on the energies around us—and on how those "external" energies will or will not influence us.

Being aware of our thoughts can help us choose consciously how we will think, interact with others, respond to external situations, and move through the world. If we have a positive outlook—focusing on love, kindness, hope, peace, joy, gratitude, and forgiveness—we will more easily draw to us others of similar perspectives and energy. If we are dwelling on negative thoughts—like fear, judgment, jealousy, hate, anger, bitterness, blame—then we are more vulnerable to attracting others and situations with this type of energy. Furthermore, if we use certain thought exercises to protect our energy, this can have a tremendous effect on how we will interact, and how we will not interact, with external forces in our day-to-day lives. This is why, in choosing our thoughts carefully, we, along with the Universe, can manifest who we will become and what our best lives can be.

Now this does *not* mean we cannot have a bad day. We all do. It also does *not* mean that we are to blame for hurtful things that may happen to us. Some of us may experience a painful loss in our lives, like the death of a loved one. It's natural to have feelings of grief and sadness during those times. Some of us are or know souls who have been born to abusive parents, have been mistreated, or experienced other hurtful or traumatic circumstances or events. Because we all have free will, there are some souls who don't learn the lessons they need to and they do the wrong thing and they hurt others. We are not responsible for the hurtful things that others do. But these hurts and challenges do become a part of our journey, and we do have the ability to choose how we respond to them. We can choose to exercise our own free will and to use our thoughts to reclaim our power and take back our lives. We can choose to learn and grow, and even teach and help others, from the difficult or challenging experiences we have endured. And we can choose to heal, in whatever way that means for us.

But what does all of this mean for our own health and well-being? For some reason it makes me think of the classic *Oprah Winfrey Show* episode in which Oprah so generously surprised each of her audience members with the gift of a brand-new Pontiac G6. "You get a car! You get a car! You get a car! Everybody gets a car!" Oprah declared with pure joy and exuberance.

Well, that's how I feel about discovering the power of thought. It means that *you* and *you* and *you* and *you* get to heal!

It means that caring for ourselves spiritually, by choosing our thoughts with intention—and conversely, *not* caring for ourselves spiritually—can have an effect not only on our spiritual and mental, but also on our emotional and physical health and well-being. It means that we can change our health, and our lives, using the power of thought.

For example, we know that an individual who is an empath can become overwhelmed with feeling and absorbing external energies—often directly through the solar plexus and heart chakras. As a result, he or she can develop symptoms like anxiety, panic, phobias, feelings of sadness or depression, digestive issues, nausea, headaches, fatigue, and over time other dis-ease. However, if the same empath uses a simple thought exercise each day to connect with spirit and "shield" the solar plexus and heart chakras, he or she will be spiritually protected and may be able to reduce or eliminate those symptoms.

As another example, some of us are repeatedly thinking of something traumatic, hurtful, unfair, or unjust that happened to us long ago. We are still replaying it in our minds, reliving and feeling the experience, getting hurt or angry all over again. There is nothing wrong with feeling hurt or sad or angry. These emotions are healthy responses to an injury, trauma, or loss. But when we hold on to them over time, when we cannot let go of that initial deep hurt, then we can become our own punishers and these thoughts and feelings can become toxic to us. In turn, this toxic thought process can lead to a block in the flow of our energy and create an imbalance in our spiritual, mental, emotional, and physical bodies, as well as our chakras. Over time, this could contribute to the development of mental, emotional, and even physical symptoms and dis-ease. In contrast, if we are aware of the hurt we are holding on to, we can choose to use thought to forgive, let the pain go, restore balance, and heal. This, in turn, can be a first step to even greater healing, greater freedom.

Indeed, while the power of thought has long been discussed in spiritual circles, its potential health benefits are also being evaluated and recognized in the medical and mental health communities. While a state of meditation is considered by many to be characterized by a mind clear of thoughts and chatter—I believe a state of spiritual awareness and connection—our thoughts can be the vehicle we use to transport us to that clear, meditative place. There are many different types and approaches to meditation, such as guided meditation, mindfulness meditation, transcendental meditation, and others. Numerous scientific studies and analyses suggest many potential health benefits of meditation, including contributing to the reduction of blood pressure levels, anxiety, depression, pain, and stress and inflammatory responsiveness. Although many reports state that more research is needed to confirm the benefits of meditation, the mere evaluation and consideration of these techniques as complementary to medical care is a positive step toward caring for the whole person in the maintenance of our health and well-being. More and more, we are seeing techniques like meditation, visualization, and integrative health services being incorporated into aspects of the healthcare system. Indeed, many of my own clients are referred to me by their medical doctors and therapists. It is my hope that, one day, the standard of care will include doctors, nurses, therapists, other healthcare professionals, and spiritual and energy healers working together, collaboratively, to provide whole care to the whole person.

Some might ask why I consider the use of thought to be a part of spiritual healing and not purely a mental or even emotional process. First, I believe that all love, light, and healing energy comes from God (the Universal Source) and flows to and through us and all else. I also believe we are by our nature spiritual beings and require spiritual connection and care. Our thoughts can be the bridge to connecting with our spiritual selves and with God, and in turn, our spiritual connection is essential to maintaining balance, health, and well-being in our thoughts and throughout our spirit-mind-heart-physical bodies.

Using a few simple tools and techniques, we can change our thoughts and change our lives. With a little intentional thinking, you too can find your way to healing, health, and the whole you.

~

CHAPTER 4

Let the Healing Begin: The Power Is in You

W HEN I BEGAN RECEIVING THOUSANDS of e-mails and calls from people around the world who were struggling with chronic anxiety, panic attacks, phobias, and other related symptoms, I was shocked. I had known that people who were empaths or had unrealized or suppressed spiritual gifts were especially susceptible to developing these symptoms, but I had no idea that there were so very many people who were suffering in this way. I was particularly saddened by the parents, calling to ask for help for their children who were living their formative years in a state of anxiety and fear. My answer to these calls for help was to reach as many as I could by phone, Skype, and webinar—and to write this book, so that others who are suffering can learn to heal, to open to and love themselves, and to be free of spiritually based anxiety and empath-related symptoms.

My hope for you is that we can let the healing begin—today. From this moment forward, you and I will be partners, walking through the steps of connecting to and caring for your spiritual self—and learning the tools you will need to begin to heal and to maintain your health, balance, and wholeness today, tomorrow, and every day thereafter. Because the power to heal is in you and the time to reach out, reach in, and love yourself is here.

As we prepare to use the power of thought and our spiritual connection to begin the healing process, let's see what spiritual healing is, what it looks like, and the steps we will take as part of this process. It's what I do and teach in one of my healing sessions.

Health and Healing: It's All a Balancing Act

For me, healing is the process of bringing one's whole self into balance, in love and light, and opening the pathway for one to be fully realized in all God meant him or her to be. Health, healing, and indeed life are all about balance. A state of health and wholeness is one of balance and flow. To heal and to maintain our health, balance is vitally important in every part of ourselves and in every area of our lives.

Honoring Ourselves: Finding Balance in the Busy-ness

First, as human beings functioning in a physical world, we need to maintain a healthy balance in our day-to-day activities, our relationships, and our energy. We need to take care of and honor ourselves as well as others. This means we need a balance between our family, work, and social lives. It means in our relationships, we need to receive as well as to give. It also means listening to that still small voice inside, the one that will guide us to our soul's purpose and our joy. I believe the flight attendants have put this in very simple, useful terms for us: *Always place the oxygen mask on yourself, before assisting others.*

One gentleman I was blessed to meet did exactly this. After feeling unhappy for some time, Christopher had come to me for a healing due to an issue with high blood pressure. He had a highly successful job in marketing. He had a brilliant career ahead of him. He had status. He had money. And he was miserable. In talking to Christopher, we discovered that, while he felt responsible for family and friends who were relying on him for financial support, all Christopher wanted was to become a police officer. Christopher and I completed the healing session, and I gave him his homework exercises to help him to continue to heal and to maintain his health and balance going forward.

Months later, I ran into Christopher at an event. He came up to me with a big hello and beaming smile, but I did not recognize him. He had lost thirty pounds, he was now a police officer, and he was happy. Christopher had listened to his still small voice, honored himself, and found his truth.

It's important to find our truth and follow our dreams, but also to do even this in a balanced and responsible way, like Christopher did. It doesn't mean that we should abruptly quit a full-time paying job so that we can work exclusively on creating our own line of jewelry when we have four kids to support. But if creating jewelry is the form of expression that calls to us, it is important to follow that dream. If we set aside time each week to honor this calling and work diligently on the creative and business aspects, we may soon be in a position to launch our own jewelry line. Or we may simply enjoy creating a beautiful work of art and sharing it with family, friends, and charitable causes. It's important, in some way, to honor our dreams and pursue our passions. And it's important to find time for ourselves. For some of us, it's as simple as being able to get to the gym or go bowling two or three times a week. As our flight attendant professionals know well, if we are depleted, we will not be of much help to others for very long. And ultimately, the more full of heart we are, the better parents, children, siblings, friends, colleagues, and citizens we will be.

Connecting to Spirit and Earth

As souls living on earth, we need to maintain a balance between the spiritual and the physical elements within us. This means we make the commitment to ourselves to develop and maintain on a regular basis our connection with both heaven and earth.

As we seek to connect with our spiritual selves, we need only to look and listen within. Through a connection with our own spiritual selves, we can access our higher selves, our spirit guides and other spiritual beings, and the Divine.

GOD. I use the name "God" to refer to the Divine, the Source, the Universe of all that is love, light, and goodness. To me, God is the consciousness of love. I also believe that the presence of God, or the Divine, resides within each of us. It is this presence and ability to connect with God that is the source of our intuition and all of our spiritual gifts, including what we sometimes call psychic, mediumship, and healing abilities.

SPIRIT GUIDES. I believe that a spirit guide is a being who exists in spirit form and has committed to watch over us, guide us, and help us to learn and to teach what we need on this earthly journey. I also believe each of us is assigned at least one spirit guide before we are born into the human life. This spirit guide is a being who has lived on the earth in the past, so that they may draw upon their experience with the human condition, including the feeling of human emotion, to help guide us. A spirit guide could be a family member or other soul who lived on earth before we did. Indeed, even highly elevated souls such as Jesus, the Blessed Mother Mary, Muhammed, Buddha, and all of the Ascended Masters once walked the earth and may be working as spirit guides for a great multitude of souls. In addition to having spirit guides who have had the human experience, I believe each of us is also assisted and guided by angels. Angels work in pure spirit form as Divine messengers of God, guiding and serving with perfect compassion (but don't be surprised if you also run into an angel or two on earth!). Some of us are able to see, hear, or feel the presence of our spirit guides and other beings in spirit form, while others of us just know they are there. Some people report feeling or knowing that a spirit guide protected them in a time of need. A car crash that should have killed them. A feeling or voice inside that said don't walk that way home today. A favorite flower that grew out of season, with no apparent explanation. The stories are endless. Whether we see, hear, or feel them or not, our spirit guides are there. And for all of us, the message is you are not alone, we are here, we are with you, we love you.

SPIRITUAL BEINGS. This includes everyone! We are all spiritual beings by nature, whether we are currently living in spirit or physical form. However, many people use the term "spiritual beings" to refer to those who are living in the spirit world. This includes God, archangels, and angels. It also includes our loved ones whose physical bodies have passed away and who are now alive and well on the other side. In connecting with our spiritual selves, we can also connect with these spiritual beings. We can communicate with them directly, or we can ask our spirit guides to help facilitate a visit for us.

HIGHER SELF. Some people refer to the higher self as simply the spiritual self, or the soul. I think of our higher self as the best or highest part of who we are. Whether that is our soul or the highest part of our soul, does anyone really know? I sometimes refer to the higher self as our "God self." If God represents the highest vibration of energy, then our higher selves represent that presence of God in each of us. Our spiritual selves, or our souls, have come to earth to learn and evolve to this higher vibration, to that of God and of love. As part of this process of evolvement, we learn to live and breathe and walk through the world from the perspective of our higher selves, in this presence of God. I believe we can all access and view the world from the perspective of our higher selves at any time. I believe we do this more and more often, for longer periods of time, as our souls learn and evolve. Until one day, we simply are one with our higher self and with God. We are love.

SPIRITUAL SELF. When I refer to the spiritual self, I am referring to the spiritual part of us, or the soul. The spiritual self is also sometimes called the spiritual body. I believe that each of us is an eternal spiritual being who lived before we were born to earth and will continue to live after our physical bodies have passed away. I also believe that our spiritual selves, or souls, may choose to take physical form, on earth or other destinations, over a multitude of lifetimes. This is the soul's way of learning, growing, and ultimately evolving to the consciousness of love.

When we begin to become more aware of and to connect spiritually to ourselves, God, and others, we must remember the need for balance here as well. When seeking to connect spiritually, balance means grounding. Grounding is a way to connect, both spiritually and physically, with the earth. Over the years, I have found that people become very excited about their ability to connect spiritually and to develop and share their spiritual gifts. Sometimes, they are so excited that they forget that grounding is equally important. Indeed, I have observed that the more and better we ground, the more quickly and more clearly our spiritual gifts tend to manifest. In the pages ahead, we will learn how to connect spiritually but also to ground, ground, ground.

The Four Bodies and Seven Main Chakras

If we remember that we are multidimensional beings—having a spiritual, mental, emotional, and physical body, along with seven main chakras helping us to connect and maintain a flow of our energy—then also essential to our health is that these bodies and chakras are in balance and our energy is flowing freely throughout our whole selves.

Dis-ease—by which I mean a disturbance in the ease and wellness of our being—can originate in any of our four bodies, and can cause or be caused by an imbalance and a block in the flow of our energy in any one of our bodies or chakras. Because we are energy and our four bodies are all part of us, part of our energy field or aura, dis-ease in any one of the four bodies can affect the other three bodies. Thus, anxiety and other symptoms or dis-ease can come from a number of different places, in a number of different ways.

Let's look at the physical body. Say a man is in a car accident and, as a result, his spinal cord is damaged. He experiences the

physical symptom of temporary paralysis. Because of this physical injury, he may also experience mental and emotional pain
such as anxiety and feelings of depression over the loss of his
mobility, medical bills, and uncertainty about his future. It's
possible he could also develop a fear or phobia of driving or riding in a car or in traffic. He may struggle spiritually, asking
himself why this happened to him, why he is here, and what his
life's purpose may be given these unforeseen circumstances.
This can be the case in varying degrees for any physical dis-
ease, from injury to infection to inherited syndromes to
environmentally related conditions to those derived from a
combination of these factors.

So too, dis-ease of the emotional body can affect the other
bodies. If we experience an emotional trauma or loss, this
could trigger a range of feelings, from hurt to anger, sadness,
shame, guilt, fear, and anxiety. If, for example, we were be-
trayed in a marriage or other relationship, we could
experience hurt, disbelief, and anger. We could experience
feelings of anxiety, shame, or hopelessness, feeling that something is wrong with us, wondering why we didn't see this
coming, and whether we will ever be able to trust in love again.
This energy moves to our mental body and can manifest as
thought forms that either help us to cope and heal or, in contrast, repeat and reinforce this pain for weeks, months, or even
years after the initial event has ended. Such an emotional injury can also cause spiritual pain, leaving us to wonder why
this happened to us and what it means. If we hold on to these
hurtful thought forms and emotions, over time, they can cause
physical stress and symptoms as well.

If we consider the mental body, we know that some of us
have been diagnosed with dis-ease such as anxiety disorders,
clinical depression, obsessive-compulsive disorder, bipolar
disorder, and many others. In some people, there is a genetic

predisposition. For some, the physical brain is impaired or is lacking in the chemicals it needs to function optimally. In others, they have suffered emotional trauma in their past that has contributed to them developing anxiety, depression, or both. Dis-ease of the mental body can, in turn, trigger additional emotional pain—causing difficulty in our moods, connections with other people, and sometimes even feelings of embarrassment or stigma. Our struggles with our mental health can also lead to physical effects. Some individuals with anxiety also have symptoms such as upset stomach, fatigue, and feeling depressed. Some people with depression report feeling physical pain along with depressive symptoms. Sadly, in some people, this type of illness can even result in their ending their physical lives. In my experience, many who have been diagnosed with mental illness also experience related spiritual suffering—sometimes feeling completely disconnected from their spiritual selves and other persons or, alternatively, living spiritually wide open, seeming "out there" or "out of it," without the appropriate protection and grounding in our earthly existence.

When we look at the spiritual body, I believe that, for many of us, the lack of awareness of or connection to and protection of our spiritual selves is a contributing factor in the development of anxiety and related dis-ease. When we stop listening to that still small voice inside, we can lose ourselves. So too, when we are empaths and we are unknowingly taking on and absorbing the negative, toxic, or unbalanced feelings and energies of others, this can lead to a disruption in the balance and flow of our energy. And when we are unaware of or deny our spiritual selves, including our intuition and related spiritual gifts, this can cause a block or a buildup of energy within us that will come out eventually, one way or another. The effects can be not only spiritual, but also mental, emotional, and physical. As we saw with our empath friends, a lack of spiritual awareness and protection can manifest as anxiety, panic attacks, phobias, feelings of sadness or depression, headaches, exhaustion (doesn't it sound exhausting?), and other symptoms or dis-ease. In our empath friend Nick, we saw that his lack of spiritual protection and recognition of his intuitive gifts was contributing to his symptoms of extreme anxiety. For Jennifer, it was this same lack of awareness that was a factor in her depression.

Another way to think about health and dis-ease and the importance of balance is to understand more about our *chakras*, which are like the energy wheels or centers of our body. Each of our seven main chakras receives and radiates energy, spinning clockwise to propel vital life-force energy I believe from the Divine—through our many other chakras and four bodies.

The seven main chakras are represented by the seven colors of the rainbow. The colors of the chakras are also reflected in our auras. As part of my gift, I am able to see these auras and therefore am able to observe the beautiful colors of the chakras present in our auric fields. When a person is healthy and balanced, the colors appear to me as bright and shimmering like gemstones—and transparent and clear, almost like Jell-O. When a person is not balanced, the colors look more dark, muddy, and solid. Each chakra corresponds with its own area of the physical body, as well as with our physical, emotional, mental, and/or spiritual states of being. Our job is to keep our chakras open, clear, and balanced in order to facilitate healing and maintain our well-being.

Whether we are referring to our four bodies, our chakras, the Universal Life Force or energy that flows through us, or the logistics of our day-to-day lives, one of the most important

A Little About Our Seven Main Chakras

The first chakra, or root chakra

- This chakra is located between the tailbone and pelvic bone.
- The first chakra is considered to be one of earth or matter, meaning it helps connect us with the earth.
- The root chakra helps to ground us. When open and in balance, it brings us feelings of safety, security, and stability.
- Of the seven main chakras, the root chakra spins at the slowest rate.
- To me, the color of the root chakra (via my observations of it in the aura) is a bright, clear, shiny ruby red. When not in balance, the color appears to me as a less transparent, darker, kind of muddy red.

The second, or sacral, chakra

- This chakra, also sometimes referred to as the spleen chakra, is located between the navel and pelvic bone.
- This is often referred to as our creative and sexual center.
- The second chakra is also one of the earth or matter, helping us to connect with the physical world.
- When open and in balance, this chakra brings us feelings of creativity, pleasure, joy, abundance, and overall wellness of being.
- This chakra spins slightly faster than the root chakra.
- In the aura, I see the color of the sacral chakra reflected as a bright, clear, shimmering orange. When not in balance, the color appears to me as darker and more opaque, kind of like a cheese-doodle orange.

The third, or solar plexus, chakra

- This chakra resides at the solar plexus, the area between the navel and breastbone. It's that spot right in the center of and just below the rib cage. Some people say just over or above the stomach.

- The third chakra is also a chakra of the earth.
- I often refer to this chakra as the "seat of intuition," because I believe much of our sense of feeling (like a gut feeling) occurs through this chakra.
- I believe this chakra is responsible for much of the type of intuition that often manifests as a "gut feeling." We can "feel" information through the solar plexus and heart chakras, and these feelings can help direct our assessments and decisions: yes or no, this way or that way, stay or go.
- In empaths who have a heightened sensitivity to the feelings and energy of other people, animals, and places—which they absorb through the solar plexus—an unprotected solar plexus chakra can lead to anxiety, panic attacks, nausea, digestive issues, tiredness, low energy, and poor stamina. This can also be the case for people who receive psychic information as "feelings" through the solar plexus or heart centers.
- This chakra spins faster than the sacral chakra.
- When reflected in the aura, I see the color of the solar plexus chakra as that of bright, clear, golden sunshine. When not in balance, it appears a darker, more opaque yellow.

The fourth chakra, also called the heart chakra

- The heart chakra is located in the center of the chest.
- I think of this chakra as the juncture of heaven and earth, the meeting of both spirit and earth chakras.
- When this chakra is open, we experience the giving and receiving of love freely, love of ourselves, and love of others.
- As with the solar plexus chakra, I believe we can also feel and absorb the feelings and energies of others through the heart chakra. For empaths and those with heightened psychic and mediumship abilities, an unprotected heart chakra also can

result in anxiety, panic attacks, feelings of sadness, and lack of self-love.

- This chakra spins faster than the solar plexus chakra.
- In the aura, I see the color associated with the heart chakra as a bright, clear neon green. I often see this as the predominant color in the auras of healers. When not in balance, the color appears as a more solid, darker, hunter green.

The fifth, or throat, chakra

- This chakra resides in the throat.
- The throat chakra is considered to be a chakra of spirit.
- When open, this chakra helps to facilitate communication, including speaking and listening. In my practice, I have found that those who have been unable to speak their own truth—including those who have heightened psychic or mediumship abilities that they have suppressed or not yet discovered—can develop symptoms such as nervousness or discomfort when speaking, dis-ease of the thyroid or tongue, neck, eating disorders, chronic sore throat, laryngitis, colds, swollen glands, and dental problems.
- The spirit chakras spin progressively faster than the lower chakras.
- When I view this chakra's color in the auric field, it appears as a bright, shimmering, turquoise blue, like the sky on a light and clear day. When not in balance, the color appears to me as a darker, more solid blue.

The sixth chakra, or third eye

- This chakra is located on the forehead, slightly above the center of the eyebrows.
- The third eye is the second chakra of spirit.
- The third eye is considered by many to be an intuitive center and responsible for clear intuitive "seeing" or vision.
- In my experience, people who have a blocked or imbalanced

third eye, or those who have a heightened sense of intuitive see-ing or knowing but are not aware of or suppress it, can experience frequent headaches, migraines, issues with vision such as eye strain and conjunctivitis, sinus issues, memory issues, and other symptoms.

- Many say the color of the third-eye chakra is indigo. When re-flected in the aura, I actually see the color as bright clear violet or a shimmering royal purple. For me, this is the predominant color I see in in the aura of people who have strong psychic or mediumship abilities. I see violet when the person's gift is still de-veloping and royal purple when their gift is more fully developed. When not in balance, the color appears to me as a darker, more solid gray-violet or gray-purple.

The seventh, or crown, chakra

- The seventh chakra is located at the very top, or crown, of the head. Some even say it resides just above the head.
- The crown chakra is a chakra of spirit.
- This chakra facilitates our connection to God or the Universal consciousness.
- When open, this chakra brings us a higher connection to all that is.
- People who have a blocked crown chakra can feel disconnected from their spiritual selves. People whose crown chakra is wide open but unprotected—or those who have a heightened sense of spiritual connection and psychic and mediumship abilities but are unaware of this or suppress them—can experience symp-toms such as anxiety, panic attacks, and frequent headaches. They can also lack grounding in the physical world, and have a difficult time staying connected to earth and their earthly life.
- Many people consider the color associated with the crown chakra to be purple or violet. For whatever reason, I see this color reflected in the aura as a bright, gleaming white. The more highly evolved the person, the whiter and brighter the color appears.

keys to healing, health, and wellness is balance. Our job is to keep our four bodies and our chakras open, aligned, and balanced, with a constant, steady flow of energy running through them. This means that we need to be aware of and care for our whole selves—yes, including our spiritual selves—to heal and to maintain a state of health and wellness. And we have lots of tools to help us do this!

Spiritual Healing: What Does It Look Like?

There are many forms of healing from the use of medications to surgical procedures, to psychotherapy, physical therapy, acupuncture, massage, different types of meditative practices, and countless others. My role is one of a spiritual healer, and my modality is that of an energy healing. Even within the practice of energy healing, there are many different approaches and techniques that are used.

While all parts of us, even our physical selves, are made of energy, I refer to the energy healing I provide as "spiritual healing" because the foundation of my work is my faith in God (or the Universal Source). I believe all healing energy originates from God, that we are all spiritual beings by nature, and that connecting with God's love, light, and healing energy can bring healing not only to the spirit, but in many cases, also to the mind, heart, and/or physical body.

When I do an energy healing, I am connecting with my higher self, my spirit guides, the archangels, and with God to facilitate the healing process. I ask God to allow me to be a channel for His gold and white light and healing energy to flow through me and into the recipient(s). I set my intention for "the highest good" of that individual and all concerned. In addition to this, I instruct those who come for healing on how to use tools such as intention, affirmation, meditation, prayer, and visualization to connect with their own spiritual or higher selves and with the Divine to help them heal, protect, ground, and balance themselves on a day-to-day basis.

While this is the approach I use, it's important to note that if you do not use the word "God," you can use whatever term works for you. Spiritual healing is not limited to those of any particular faith. It is open to those of all religions as well as to those who do not practice any particular religion. Because we are all spiritual beings, all souls, the purpose is for you to become aware of and to be present with your spiritual self, the part of you that is connected to the Universal consciousness of goodness, to all that is light and love. I call that God.

Since I began my work as a spiritual healer, people have come to me for help with all different types of dis-ease. For those whose suffering is spiritually based, the effect of spiritual healing can be almost immediate. Many empaths who have come with debilitating anxiety and panic attacks report feeling calm, peaceful, and lighter even before they leave the session. Many call or email after their appointments, telling me that their anxiety is much better or completely resolved. For those whose symptoms were spiritually based but manifested physically (such as chronic fatigue, weakness, headache), the healing effect may take a little longer. In addition, because all four of our bodies are energy and are connected, spiritual healing can have a benefit in addressing not only dis-ease that originates in the spiritual body, but also in the mental, emotional, and even physical bodies. Just as imbalance and dis-ease can move to our different bodies, so too can healing. I have been humbled to witness countless individuals make complete recoveries from all sorts of "physical" dis-ease—from inherited syndromes to neurological disorders to autoimmune disease to cancer.

While I believe everyone can benefit from spiritual healing, it's important to know that spiritual healing does not always result in a complete recovery of all four bodies in all people. I learned early on that healing is different for different people at different times in their journeys. Depending on the soul's agreement with God, and on the person's free-will choices, the effect of the healing may come in the form of spiritual, mental, emotional, and/or physical healing. It may indeed manifest as a complete physical recovery, alleviation or complete resolution of symptoms, new opening to and love for one's self, a reconnection with loved ones, or for some, even a sense of peace and comfort before passing.

I believe some of us, perhaps the brave among us, have a soul's agreement with God to live with the challenge of a disease in order to learn and to teach certain lessons, to help raise our own consciousness and that of others. I believe some of us have a soul's agreement to live through certain difficult experiences or events so that we may be challenged, for the purpose of our learning and that of others. For some of us, our soul's destiny, along with our free-will choice, may mean that healing manifests as a complete and total restoration of the spiritual, mental, emotional, and physical bodies. For others, like poet and peacemaker Mattie Stepanek who passed away of dysautonomic mitochondrial myopathy at age thirteen, our soul's agreement with God may mean that we are balanced, healthy, and whole in spirit, mind, and heart, but our bodies are meant to remain vulnerable in order to emphasize and amplify the lessons we are here to teach or learn. Individuals like these, especially those who are with us for such a short while, are special souls who deliver tremendous gifts of love and wisdom in the precious little time that they have on earth. And of course, at some point in our human lives, each of us will shed our physical shells and return to the fully spiritual beings that we are and always will be. This is our earthly sojourn.

While healing may be different for different people at different points in their journey, there is no reason to accept a state of dis-ease. There is always some type of healing to benefit the recipient and others. And in my experience, many individuals who present with unexplained anxiety, panic attacks, phobias, irrational fears, feelings of sadness or depression, fatigue, digestive issues, frequent headaches, and other empath-related symptoms have a spiritual component to this dis-ease. I have seen thousands use simple spiritual healing, protection, and maintenance exercises and find their way to healing, wholeness, and a life free of these symptoms.

Our Doctors, Nurses, and Therapists

Many people ask me some variation of this question: "If spiritual healing and care can help maintain our health, balance, and well-being, then why do we need to see our doctor, therapist, or other health professional?" And many others ask me: "If spiritual healing requires faith, then I can't see my doctor, therapist, or other health professional. If I do, won't that mean that I don't have faith in God and in His healing power?"

So here's the thing. Every person requires care of their spiritual, mental, emotional, and physical selves. I view spiritual healing as something to be done in collaboration with, not instead of, medical and psychosocial care. This includes medical care when you feel sick, and preventive and maintenance care to keep you feeling well.

If you are suffering with anxiety, I highly recommend that you see a trusted doctor and perhaps therapist to help identify and treat any physical, mental, or emotional basis for your symptoms. For many people, medications, psychotherapy, and/or other therapy may be able to help alleviate anxiety and related symptoms. Like any other line of work, medicine is not perfect and not all health professionals can help every single patient every single time. In some cases, an illness is misdiagnosed. In other cases, unnecessary medications are given or the medical intervention is not working. It's important to ensure that the doctor or therapist you choose is respected and able to provide state-of-the-art care in his or her area of expertise. It's also important that he or she listens and cares about you and your well-being. We all know the difference between someone who cares and someone who doesn't. If your doctor or therapist has not been able to help you or your loved one, I would recommend you consider seeking a second opinion from another doctor or therapist.

In addition to medical and psychosocial care, I advise that you also participate in spiritual healing and care, because I think it may help you a great deal and, quite possibly, very quickly. After starting a spiritual healing regimen, I recommend that you continue to see your doctor or therapist as you usually would. This is important: Please do not reduce or discontinue any medications or therapies without talking with your doctor first. When you visit with your doctor, and if you are feeling better, you can discuss with him or her at that time whether tapering off or discontinuing a medication or other treatment may be right for you. If he or she agrees, you can do this under his or her medical supervision, to ensure that you do it in the way that is healthiest and safest for you.

In terms of faith, I have an unmovable faith in God and in His healing power. But I don't believe that you have to use the term "God" to be healed. You simply have to accept that you are a part of a greater Universal consciousness of goodness and agree to receive the healing. However, if you do have a strong faith in God, as I do, who is to say that God did not also send the doctor or the nurse or the therapist to help you?

For me, it brings to mind the old story about the man in the flood:

A man was trapped in his house during a flood. He began praying to God to rescue him. The water started to rise in his house. His neighbor urged him to leave and offered him a ride to safety. The man yelled back, "I am waiting for God to save me." The neighbor drove off in his pickup truck.

The man continued to pray. As the water began rising in his house, he had to climb up to the roof. A boat came by with some people heading for safe ground. They yelled at the man to grab a rope they were ready to throw and take him to safety. He told them that he was waiting for God to save him. They shook their heads and moved on.

The man continued to pray, believing with all his heart that he would be saved by God. The flood waters continued to rise. A helicopter flew by and a voice came over a loudspeaker offering to lower a ladder and take him off the roof. The man waved the helicopter away, shouting back that he was wait-ing for God to save him. The helicopter left. The flooding water came over the roof and caught him up and swept him away. He drowned.

When he reached heaven, he asked, "God, why did you not save me? I believed in you with all my heart. Why did you let me drown?" God replied, "I sent you a pickup truck, a boat, and a helicopter and you refused all of them. What more could I do?"

This is exactly the way I feel about doctors, nurses, therapists, and other health professionals! When my mother was diagnosed with metastatic breast cancer and experienced a miraculous result after a session with a local spiritual healer (that was how I learned about spiritual healing!), she still continued to see her oncologist for a time. When my husband was diagnosed with cancer, he saw the specialists necessary to provide him with the best care available. When I needed surgery, I went to a surgeon and I had surgery. I am grateful to these medical professionals and for their years of education and the expertise and service they provide. I believe our doctors and other health professionals, too, are healers. They, too, are partners in our care. We need to utilize their abilities fully and honor and thank them for what they do. We are all working together to foster health and wellness.

The Power Is in You

As I shared with you earlier, way back in the beginning of my healing work, my sessions consisted of an energy healing alone. Many people diagnosed with all kinds of dis-ease seemed to experience a complete and permanent healing, and I was honored to be able to be a part of their return to balance and wellness. But I also began to realize that, for some individuals, a one-time energy healing performed by a third party was not sufficient to maintain long-term health, balance, and wholeness. Especially for some who had suffered with long-term chronic symptoms, they would experience a significant or even complete healing effect, and then, after a few months, their symptoms would begin to resurface.

Over time, I learned that this "relapse" of sorts was happening because each individual needs to own and participate in his or her own healing, health, and wellness. Part of this participation is a willingness to work to identify and address the factors that contributed to the underlying symptoms or disease in the first place. The other part is a commitment to doing the homework to "maintain" the healing—to using our connection with spirit and the power of thought to protect, ground, balance, and heal—not only on the first day, but every day after. Especially for empaths, we know that an ongoing practice of spiritual protection and grounding is essential to do each and every day. Finally, any spiritual gifts that are hidden, unrealized, or otherwise being suppressed must be recognized and accepted. As I said in the beginning, our healing starts with loving ourselves—our whole selves.

Because my clients are such good teachers, I was able to learn these lessons and alter my healing sessions, so that the individual and I are working in partnership in their healing and spiritual care. As a result, my healing sessions quickly came to include five steps, all of which I will be sharing with you in the chapters ahead. These steps include the following:

- Daily surround, ground, and shield exercises for spiritual protection and balance
- Identification and release (using forgiveness) of any negative thoughts and feelings related to underlying hurts, injuries, losses, or circumstances that may be contributing to or causing symptoms or dis-ease
- Daily thought exercises to help raise our vibration— to elevate our thoughts in order to maintain health and balance and to manifest our best lives
- An energy healing: channeling God's gold and white light, love, and healing energy to balance, ground, and heal in spirit-mind-heart-body for the highest good

- Tools to help us connect with, open to, and accept our
spiritual self and intuitive gifts

The tools we will use as part of these steps to spiritual healing and health are quick, simple exercises that anyone can do.
These exercises build upon what I like to call our superpowers
of Intention, Imagination, and Intuition.

Our Superpowers

As we begin our journey toward healing and wholeness,
it's important to understand the fundamental role and power
of our Intention, Imagination, and Intuition.

INTENTION. Intention is the use of our thoughts to set forth
in advance what we intend, or what our goal is to become or
manifest. When setting our intention, we may do so at many
different levels: for our lives (such as to live with integrity and
kindness), for each day, for a project, or for a specific person,
task, or situation. Many of us have heard the phrase, "The
road to hell is paved with good intentions." I do not believe
this. I believe if our intention is of love and light, then regard-
less of the consequence or outcome, we have contributed to
the good. It's possible that we, being human, may miscalculate
the true need of a situation or mess up the execution of our intention, but if the intention is pure, I believe it will serve the
greater good, even if this is not evident to us at the time.

This does, however, demonstrate the need to be very careful with our intentions. When I set my intention to facilitate
a healing for someone, for example, I do so for that person's
highest good and let God make the determination as to what
that may be. I am careful not to limit my own or anyone else's
potential or healing by being limited in my intention.

Setting our intention is powerful. If we do not set our intention, we live passively, taking whatever comes our way. When we mindfully set our intention for the highest good, all of the Universe gets behind it. All of the Universe conspires to support us and the goodness we are intending. As part of the healing process, we will need to set our intention in a conscious, proactive, and deliberate way to direct our thoughts, our words and actions, our healing, and ultimately our lives. Our intention is the cornerstone of all thought exercises.

IMAGINATION. We all know how to imagine. We can use our thoughts to imagine all kinds of things, from the children we would like to have someday, to successes in our careers, to talking just one more time to a loved one who has passed. In our imagination, we can use all of our human senses: vision, sound, taste, smell, and touch. But our imagination is much more powerful than many people realize. While our society values the role of imagination in creative ventures, it can sometimes devalue this super power in other areas as something fanciful, pretend, or not real. As we know, the imagination can spark creative ideas and innovations, some of them revolutionary or even lifesaving. I also believe that the imagination can be the bridge to our spiritual selves and spiritual gifts. Indeed, our thought exercises will utilize the power of imagination to start us on the road to healing and to finding and developing our own sense of intuition.

INTUITION. We talked about our intuition as that still small voice inside, the sense or communication that comes through our connection with our spiritual self and with God that guides us in our day-to-day lives and in our soul's destiny. We know that each one of us possesses our own unique gift of intuition, and that some of us may have an exceptionally heightened sense of intuition and not even know it. Whatever our intuitive abilities may be, we can all benefit from becoming more aware of and strengthening this powerful gift. We can use our intention, imagination, and our current intuitive ability to guide us in strengthening our spiritual connection and developing this power even further. Like a muscle, the more we become aware of it, the more we use it, the stronger it will become. In turn, I believe it's important to do this by taking the needed steps to spiritual healing and care, to ensure we discover and develop our intuition and related spiritual gifts in a healthy, balanced manner—and thus further promote our healing and wholeness.

OUR THREE SUPERPOWERS form the foundation for the thought tools that we will use throughout the steps in our healing process. Utilizing the three I's, we will use specific techniques to help us to connect with our spiritual selves, protect ourselves spiritually, balance and ground, let go of past hurts, raise our vibration, and open to and develop our own spiritual gifts—and ultimately to heal.

A Few of Our Thought Tools and Techniques

We know that thoughts become things. Using a few simple tools, our thoughts can become our healing and the realization of our whole and true selves. A few of our thought exercises will include affirmation, intention, meditation, prayer, and visualization.

AFFIRMATION. An affirmation is a positive statement that we say to ourselves. It can be used to help us reframe our own thoughts about ourselves in a more positive way, to encourage ourselves, and to manifest the desires of our hearts and souls. An affirmation is stated in the present tense, in a way that indicates that our desire is already the case (such as "I am healthy, balanced, and whole in spirit, mind, heart, and body"). It can be used alone, or as part of another exercise such as visualization or meditation. It can be said silently, verbally, in writing, or even as part of a song or chant.

BREATHING OR BREATH WORK. Okay, technically breath work may not be considered a thought exercise, but it's an essential tool to use along with our thought exercises. And we do need to think to remember to use it! There are many different breathing techniques that can be used, often to help us to relax and to focus our attention on the present moment. When doing so, it is important to breathe in through the nose, all the way into the belly, out through the mouth . . . with the abdomen rising and falling with each inhalation and exhalation. Breathing techniques can be used alone or with other exercises such as visualization and meditation. They can also be very helpful in ending a panic attack, by focusing on our breathing and mindfully changing from anxious shallow breaths to deep abdominal breathing.

INTENTION. While Intention is one of our superpowers and the cornerstone of all of our thought exercises, I also use the term "intention" to refer to a specific type of exercise. I use this term to refer to an exercise where we simply use our thoughts and energy to "intend" something to be. An intention can be sent silently or expressed verbally, in writing, or other expression.

MEDITATION. There are many different definitions of meditation and many ways to meditate. Merriam-Webster defines to "meditate" as "to engage in mental exercise (such as concentration on one's breathing or repetition of a mantra for the purpose of reaching a heightened level of spiritual awareness." I think of meditation as listening to God. Often, the purpose of meditation is to develop a closer connection with our spiritual selves, spiritual guides, and God. Another characterization describes the purpose of meditation as to simply be in a nonjudgmental state in the present moment. To do this, we use the power of thought to take us to a place in which our minds become clear of thoughts and chatter, and we can experience the quiet stillness of the spiritual connection. Sometimes, the purpose of a meditation can be very specific, such as forgiving, grounding, balancing the chakras, or doing an energy healing. The techniques used to reach this state of quiet meditation are many. They can include anything from focusing the mind on a breathing technique to using an audio "guided meditation," sitting in silence, looking into a candle flame, listening to meditation music, sitting in nature, or using visualization to help us use our imagination as the bridge to a meditative state.

PRAYER. A prayer is a mode of communication with God. If meditation is listening to God, then prayer is talking to God. A prayer typically is sent by us to God, and can be a request, thank-you, praise, or any other message we wish to convey. It can be said in our own words or visual images or as a more formal or established religious prayer or song. A prayer can be carried out silently, verbally, or in writing. It can be done alone or as part of a group.

VISUALIZATION. This is a technique that uses our imagination to create an idea or mental picture in our mind, often to create or manifest what we want. For example, if an empath is experiencing anxiety or panic attacks, he may wish to visualize or envision a vest of armor covering and protecting his solar plexus and heart chakras from front to back (see chapter 5). If an individual experiences obsessive and intrusive thoughts, she may wish to envision in her mind's eye a picture of her mind as a crystal-clear blue lake with no ripples. It is okay if we cannot see the picture, as long as we have the intention. Anytime we are imagining or envisioning a picture or image in our mind's eye, we are using visualization. Visualization can be used alone or with other exercises, such as affirmation, intention, or meditation.

IF YOU ARE up for a partnership, I would like to offer you the same steps, the same guidance and simple tools I use in my healing sessions to help you achieve and maintain healing, health, and wholeness in your own life. What I do, you can do for yourself. The power is in *you*.

CHAPTER 5

Surround, Ground, and Shield: Activating Your Spiritual Defense System

WHEN I BEGIN A HEALING session for someone with anxiety, there are times when the person is so anxious or disconnected or fatigued that they are unable to participate in their own healing at that initial moment. These individuals are almost always empaths who are being inundated and overwhelmed by the energies around them. They may be too anxious, jittery, or restless to think and speak about their symptoms or experiences. Sometimes they may be tuned out or shut down, unable to connect or even maintain eye contact. This is why, for people who are experiencing anxiety, I start my healing sessions with the surround, ground, and shield exercises.

First, I gently suggest, "Would you like to put that pillow in front of you?" Oftentimes, sitting with the pillow placed in front of their abdomen will alleviate their anxiety enough that we can proceed with a discussion of why they are here and what symptoms they are experiencing. Just like that! This is because the use of physical objects can help protect those of us who are empaths by shielding and protecting the solar plexus and heart—the two chakra centers that I believe are usually the most involved in feeling, taking in, and absorbing the energy of others (including people, animals, places, and spiritual beings). The pillow is essentially acting as a "shield." This same effect can be achieved by placing pets or items like our pocketbooks in front of us, wearing a big sweater or a vest around our chest and solar plexus area, or for a baby, using swaddling blankets or clothing. Many empaths will do this without even being aware of it, by folding their arms or bringing up their knees in front of their abdomen and chest.

It is this same concept that we will utilize in practicing our three main thought exercises, or intentions, to help protect and ground us. I call these exercises Surround, Ground, and Shield. These exercises are helpful for all human beings, to ensure our overall spiritual care and well-being on an ongoing basis. For people suffering with chronic anxiety, panic, irrational fears, and other empath-related symptoms, they are essential. These exercises work to protect and ground our energy, thus helping to minimize or alleviate what I refer to as "spiritually based symptoms." These are symptoms that are derived through our nature as spiritual beings and, for empaths, at least in part from a heightened sense of intuition, contributing to a heightened perception and sensitivity to the energies around them, whether the energies be those of people, animals, objects, places, or spiritual beings or information. Interestingly, I have also seen the surround, ground, and shield exercises help in alleviating other conditions, and sometimes even reduce some of the empath-related sensitivities to physical stimuli such as light, sounds, and fragrances. When performed daily, these same exercises also will help you to maintain your spiritual care and prevent symptoms from occurring.

This approach is similar to the one our physicians, nurses, and even our grandmothers refer to when they advise us that "an ounce of prevention is worth a pound of cure." They are telling us that it is worthwhile to be proactive in maintaining our physical health to reduce the risk of imbalance and dis-ease in the future. Physically, this may mean avoiding certain stressors, toxins, and carcinogens—like tobacco, harmful chemicals, too much alcohol, or overexposure to the sun. It may mean trying to watch what we eat, and maintaining a healthy body weight and level of physical activity. We may also have an annual medical checkup; keep an eye on our blood pressure, sugar, and cholesterol levels; and undergo the recommended cancer screenings. These are measures we take to avoid the things that are not good for us, build ourselves up and maintain our physical health and well-being, and actually prevent dis-ease before it starts. It's wonderful to have so many tools in our toolbox to help keep ourselves physically healthy and well.

So too, the first step in caring for ourselves spiritually is to apply similar protective and maintenance measures—a kind of spiritual defense system—to our spiritual selves. To protect and maintain our spiritual health, we need to ensure that we do not leave ourselves open to negative, toxic, unbalanced, or unwanted energies. Furthermore, we need to ensure that our own energy is grounded and balanced so that we are not over-whelmed or adversely impacted by the various energies around us.

Because we are all spiritual beings, all energy, we are con-stantly moving and working to ground and balance our own energy and that of the Universe through our spiritual, mental, emotional, and physical bodies. We are also constantly interacting and connecting with the energy all around us—from other people, animals, the earth, and the spiritual world. While much of this energy is positive, some can be negative, toxic, unbalanced, or simply unwanted. If we are not spiritually protected, grounded, and balanced ourselves, we are at the mercy of the energies around us. Basically, if we are not protected, any energy could be felt and absorbed and, further, spiritual beings with negative energy could even see an opportunity to follow us around. So too, if we are not grounded, we can be subject to "blowing in the wind" with whatever energies come our way. Being inundated with and absorbing these energies can result in imbalance and eventually can contribute to the manifestation of symptoms and dis-ease in our system. This can be true for all of us, and is especially the case for empaths.

But here's the best news ever. Just as we have tools to protect our physical health, we have tools to protect our spiritual well-being. Thoughts become things. Through our thoughts, we can connect and protect ourselves spiritually, we can ground and balance, and we can heal and maintain a state of health and healing. Using just a few simple thought exercises, we can activate our spiritual defense system and put an end to unwanted external interference and related symptoms.

Surround, Ground, and Shield Exercises

Let's get started with learning how to use our three-step spiritual defense system—our surround, ground, and shield exercises—to protect, ground, and balance ourselves. While these three exercises are designed for you to do each and every day, for protection and maintenance, they are also an essential first step for those of you who are experiencing spiritually

Exercise 1: Surround

The first exercise is an intention that is done by thought, with or without visualization. It is designed to help you connect to God and push negative energy away from your energy field.

- By thought, simply state silently or aloud, "God (or Universe), surround me in a bubble of your white light and protection."
- While you think these words, you can also use thought to visualize or picture yourself surrounded by this bubble of God's white light. But if you can't picture it, it's okay. You don't have to see it or even feel it. Just call it into being, saying the words by thought. That's it.
- This exercise takes about two seconds to complete.

based symptoms *right now*. Doing the surround, ground, and shield exercises *now* can help minimize or alleviate these symptoms and make it easier for you to engage in the other important healing steps in the chapters to come. These exercises are simple, easy, don't cost a thing, and take no more than ten seconds in total to complete. Shall we give them a try?

The surrounding exercise is the first of three exercises, to be performed together at least once each and every day. It is followed by the grounding and shielding exercises, and can be used multiple times a day as needed (morning, bedtime, before going to work or school, before a big meeting or event). This exercise helps to strengthen your connection with God and God's protection, and will get stronger over time with each use.

Because we are both spiritual and human beings, this and other grounding exercises are designed to help connect us to

Exercise 2: Ground

The second exercise is also an intention, to be used with or without visualization. It is designed to help you connect with Mother Earth, ground you here in the physical world, and thus create balance with the spiritual and physical.

- By thought, imagine three cords or roots of God's white light, extending vertically from each of your feet and your tailbone, like a tripod, deep into the center of the earth.
- Like the roots of a big tree, the light then spreads out horizontally, locking in and anchoring you solidly into the center of the earth.
- While doing this, you can also feel the energy of the earth, healing, soothing, and ultimately grounding you.
- As you do this, you can also use thought to visualize the roots of God's white light, securing you into the earth. But if you can't picture or feel it, it's okay. Just call it into being by thought.
- This grounding exercise takes about five seconds to complete.

earth and thus maintain a healthy balance and flow in our spiritual, mental, emotional, and physical bodies. I cannot tell you how many people I see who are highly spiritually aware and connected, extremely gifted, advanced in meditation and other spiritual practices, full of love and light. Yet, they do not ground themselves and they end up with anxiety, panic, headaches, fatigue, and other symptoms. Don't forget about grounding. If you live on earth, it's important. This grounding exercise should be performed at least once a day (more as needed), right after the surrounding exercise.

There are many other types of shields you can use (see below), depending on your personal preference. You can use whichever shielding tool works best for you, as long as you cover both your solar plexus and heart areas from front to back.

Exercise 3: Shield

The third exercise is also an intention, again done with or without visualization. It is designed to protect your solar plexus and heart chakras from negative, toxic, unbalanced, or otherwise unwanted energies.

- By thought, imagine wrapping yourself in a big shield, around your chest and upper abdomen area from front to back. I recommend imagining a vest of armor, like the one that Archangel Michael is often depicted wearing, covering you from heart to waist, from front to back. The vest fits over the shoulders, but it has no collar, no sleeves, and is not cumbersome. If you prefer another type of vest, you can imagine putting on a bulletproof vest, like a police officer may wear.
- The vest fits you perfectly and it is impenetrable to all outside energies that are negative, toxic, unbalanced, or unwanted.
- As you do this, you can also visualize the vest in your mind's eye, but it's okay if you cannot picture it. It's all about intention.
- The shield exe rcise takes about two to three seconds to complete.

This shielding exercise is used to prevent your solar plexus and heart chakras from taking in and absorbing unwanted external energies, thereby reducing the anxiety and other symptoms these energies can cause. The shield exercise should be done at least once a day, directly after the surround and ground exercises. It can be reapplied throughout the day as needed, particularly before challenging situations or going into crowded areas such as work, school, or a social event.

The shield exercise has evolved over time, as I have worked to develop simpler, quicker, more effective options to help protect empaths from absorbing unwanted external energies. I initially learned some exercises to protect and ground from my own teacher Holly, who was instrumental in my journey to become more spiritually aware. Holly initially introduced the idea of protecting our energy by giving us an exercise to "close down" our chakras (the body's energy wheels or centers) after our spiritual awareness class each day. This was because, after working intensively to open ourselves spiritually and develop our intuitive gifts, she did not want us to leave class "wide open" and vulnerable to unwanted energies. Holly's approach was to teach us to envision the seven main chakras as flowers that we would close up, in order to close and protect the chakras. She also offered us another version of this exercise, instructing us to picture each of the seven chakras with a steel door that we would shut tight before leaving class. This is something that I did after each of our classes, and I never had an issue. However, I did not understand at the time the connection between empaths, anxiety, and a heightened sense of intuition or sensitivity to external energies. I also only thought of this exercise as a protective measure after doing intuitive work. I did not consider this type of protection as something that may be needed on a day-to-day, preventive basis.

When I began working with my own clients and students, I started seeing more and more individuals who were experiencing symptoms—like feeling overwhelmed, inundated, and starting to see some anxiety—in certain places or situations (like crowds, hospitals) in their day- to-day lives. Over time, I began recommending the flower petal and steel door exercises to my clients and students, to be used preventively on a daily basis. As I began to learn more about the connection between empaths, their heightened perception and sensitivity to energy, and began to see more and more people with anxiety, I began to develop an exercise that could be used more quickly, more easily, and if needed, more frequently. I began teaching my clients and students to envision switching off a light switch with the intention to close and protect the chakras. In addition, one of my students, Jonathan Berardi, came up with another technique he called the zipper method, for this purpose. The zipper method is used by thinking of or visualizing the seven main chakras along the spine, and then thinking of a zipper being closed from the tailbone up and over the crown, zipping up all seven chakras.

All of these techniques (especially the zipper) worked well for my clients and students, but I still wondered if I could develop a tool that was simpler, quicker, and easier to teach. Indeed, this became a top priority for me after I appeared on the *Long Island Medium* and became absolutely inundated with calls and e-mails pouring in, most from people who were empaths suffering desperately with chronic anxiety, panic, phobias, the whole constellation of related symptoms.

One day, I found myself on Skype with a mother from the southern United States who was describing to me the debilitating anxiety and fear with which her nine-year-old son was living. It was heartbreaking. As I tried to explain to her the different thought exercises that her son could try to help protect himself and hopefully alleviate his symptoms, she asked if I could relay this information to him directly. As she went to bring her son to the computer, I didn't know how I was going to explain chakras and energy and light switches and zippers to a child. I asked God to please give me a simpler technique that I could teach easily and would be accessible and helpful to a child. In my mind's eye, I literally saw a vision of a championship wrestling belt. It was perfect! It was an image that anyone, even a child, could quickly and easily understand and apply. It was also a more targeted approach, aimed at protecting the solar plexus chakra, the energy center I had come to realize was most vulnerable in feeling and absorbing external unwanted energies. I explained to the boy that I wanted him to use his imagination to visualize putting on a championship wrestling belt, right around his upper abdomen (right over his solar plexus), each and every day. And this was the beginning of the more targeted shield exercise I teach today. The boy began to use the belt exercise and immediately began to feel better. Since that time, countless adults and children have used the belt, or some version of it (for younger children, I often ask them to imagine a super hero utility belt), and have found it highly effective in reducing their empath-related symptoms.

My shield exercise evolved even further when I observed in my practice that the heart chakra could also be a point of entry for many empaths to feel, take in, and absorb external energies. In a related discussion, one of my students noted that she had been imagining the use of a vest of armor, like the one St. Michael wears. Since that time, I have added the use of the vest, providing coverage from heart to waist, to our toolkit to protect both the solar plexus and heart chakras from these energies and thus the empath from developing the related symptoms.

Today, I advise my clients and students to use the vest of armor as part of their shielding exercise. If the vest of armor is not enough and you still find yourself experiencing anxiety, try both the vest of armor and the zipper method together. This works for most people, but by all means, add the belt, light switch, or any other of the shield exercises that you find helpful. I have some students who use them all! Importantly, the shield exercise works to block or filter out energies that are negative, toxic, unbalanced, or simply unwanted. The shield does *not* block our intuitive abilities.

It is important to remember that in addition to using our thought exercises, we can also use physical objects or clothing to help shield the solar plexus and heart areas. I once had a client who came to me after she had retired from the police department and had since developed terrible chronic anxiety. After talking with her, it was clear to me that she was an empath. After discussing this with her, including the absorption of energies through the heart and solar plexus chakras, we discovered what had suddenly triggered her symptoms of anxiety. As it turns out, she had worn a bulletproof vest every day on the police force. When she retired, she stopped wearing the bulletproof vest and promptly developed the anxiety. She was able to alleviate her symptoms by using the surround, ground, and shield thought exercises.

Finally, for those who feel like they need additional protection, grounding, and balancing, I highly recommend starting with my Universal White Light Meditation. This guided meditation takes a little longer than the very quick surround, ground, and shield exercises, but it is highly effective for those who are able to devote more time (about thirteen to fifteen minutes) to spiritual connection, protection, grounding, and balance. Please note that this meditation contains the Lord's Prayer (Our Father), which many consider to be a universal prayer of protection. I believe this prayer can be used by people of all faiths and backgrounds, but if you prefer, please feel free to use a prayer from your own faith or belief system instead.

For this, and all the meditations in this book, you may want to have someone read it to you, or make a recording yourself to play back as you meditate.

Universal White Light Meditation

The meditation you are about to experience is designed to help you surround and protect yourself with God's white light and healing energy... and to teach you to ground and balance your physical, emotional, mental, and spiritual bodies.

- I would like you to begin by sitting in a comfortable space or perhaps lying down... and begin by breathing through your nose, into your abdomen to the count of four, holding your breath for four, and blowing it out your mouth for four... and again, all the way into your belly... hold it... and blow it out your mouth for four... and one last time breathing all the way in... hold it and blow it out your mouth for four...
- Our Father who art in heaven hallowed be Thy name, Thy kingdom come, Thy will be done, on earth as it is in heaven. Give us this day our daily bread and forgive us our trespasses, as we forgive those who trespass against us and lead us not into temptation but deliver us from evil, for Thine is the kingdom, the power and the glory forever and ever, Amen...
- I would like you to imagine now, a beam of God's white light coming in through the top of

your head, through the very center of your crown chakra, filling your brain with God's white light and protection…

⇀ Imagine now or feel this light going into the center of your forehead, into your third eye and expanding it with the knowledge of the Universe…

⇀ I'd like you to imagine this light or feel this light going into your ears now and opening them up to hear your guidance, into your face, and your jaw, into your throat chakra, across your neck and shoulders, down your upper arms, through your elbows, into your forearms your wrists, your hands, and your fingers.

⇀ Imagine now or feel this light going into your heart chakra, filling your heart and your lungs with God's white light and protection… Going into your solar plexus now, below your rib cage, and into your spleen chakra, below and behind your navel. Feel this light filling every fiber and every cell of your body.

⇀ Imagine this light now going into your hips and your pelvic area, into your tailbone, which is your root chakra, through your buttocks and thighs, into your knees, your calves, your ankles, feet and toes. I'd like you to imagine now three strands of white light, one coming from the bottom of each of your feet and one coming from your tailbone.

⇀ Imagine these strands of light shooting through the floor all the way down to the very center of Mother Earth, grounding you to the earth like the roots of a tree. While at the same time pulling God's white light through the top of your head, pushing out all gray negativity into the center of the earth. Draining all gray negativity, dis-ease, and imbalance into the center of the earth.

⇥ All negativity from your physical body, all physical pain, all dis-ease and all discomfort, leaving your bodies now and draining down into the center of the earth.

⇥ Imagine, or feel this negativity leaving your emotional body. All the emotional pain of loss and disappointment down into the center of the earth. Just imagine it leaving your body…

⇥ From your mental body now, releasing all negative thought forms into the earth, all the angers, fears, the anxieties, the judgments and expectations, letting them go now into the earth, simply by thought…

⇥ And from your spiritual body now, releasing all things that are not God-like, all your ego being released into the earth.

⇥ And when all negativity has left your body, I want you to imagine gathering up all that negativity that was sent into the earth and transmuting, transforming all that negativity into magnificent white light…and allow that light now to shoot back up through your feet and through your tailbone, straight up your spine, filling you and encasing you in God's white light.

⇥ Imagine that light now, shooting back up through your crown chakra, at the very top center of your head, all the way back up to spirit,

> connecting you firmly to spirit and earth and
> then showering you in a waterfall of white light,
> protection, healing energy, and love...
> ⇁ And simply now, by closing your hands into a
> fist and slowly, gently, opening your eyes and
> coming back into the space where you began.
> Knowing that you are better for having done
> this.*

For Children and Other Loved Ones

The three-step surround, ground, and shield exercises are
simple and easy for most of us to complete. However, if you
have children or other loved ones who are not able to complete these exercises on their own (including some
individuals diagnosed with autism spectrum disorder), there
are things you can do to help them. And if children are old
enough and able to participate, there are ways to teach these
exercises in a way that is nonthreatening and maybe even fun.
For children, you may find these exercises particularly useful
before they leave for school and at bedtime to help them sleep
better. They should be done at least once each and every day,
as part of the child's routine—and then used further as
needed before birthday parties, school events, playgrounds,
or other crowded areas.

---

* This meditation can be done daily or as often as needed. You can also find this
  guided meditation on "Guided Meditations with Pat Longo" on iTunes, Amazon, and other digital platforms.

SURROUND. For the surround exercise, after you do this for yourself, simply set the same intention on your loved one's behalf. State, "God, surround <<NAME>> in a bubble of your white light and protection." At the same time, imagine him or her surrounded in the bubble of light. If you are doing this for an infant, you can also imagine bringing the child into your own bubble of light and protection, as well.

GROUND. After you complete the grounding intention for yourself, you can pray and imagine the same thing for your loved one. If he or she will permit it, you can even touch his or her hand, arm, or shoulder while you do the exercise. If the person is old enough, you can also try playing a guided meditation of the surrounding and grounding process for him or her (Universal White Light Meditation).

SHIELD. For the shield exercise, make sure you do this for yourself first. To help others, there are a few different options. If the child is an infant, it can be helpful to physically wrap him or her in swaddling clothing that includes coverage of the heart and solar plexus. You can also imagine the vest, wrapping around your child. If the child is a toddler or school-age, you can simply make a fun game of "pretend," imagining themselves wrapping up in their super hero cape, princess cape, or angel wings (covering the solar plexus and heart chakras, front and back) in the mornings and before school or other social outings. Some may like to add the super hero utility belt at the solar plexus along with their capes, vests, or wings. Young children don't need to and shouldn't understand the need for spiritual protection. You can make up whatever fantastic super hero belt or shield story that works to enthuse and empower your child. As long as they are able to "make-believe" that they are placing this shield device all the way around their heart and solar plexus area, front and back, this will have the desired effect.

Other Protective Measures

When tending to our spiritual protection, it's important to consider our environment as well as our spiritual-mental-emotional-physical selves. This includes clearing of any negativity from the space and objects around us—and being prepared to oust a more stubborn negative energy, in the rare event that this is ever needed.

ENERGY CLEARING. Some souls, both in human form and spirit form, can have negative or toxic energy. Negative energies can attach themselves not only to people, but to animals, objects, and spaces. These spiritual hitchhikers can simply follow us, a family member, or a guest right into our home. Sometimes they can take up residence in a physical space. When a spiritual hitchhiker attaches itself to us or our space, this energy can affect our own thoughts, feelings, moods, and even physical states.

For this reason, I recommend clearing your home or other space around you and your loved ones regularly. Every three months is usually sufficient, or if things suddenly seem chaotic or out of balance in your home, repeat the clearing as needed. In addition, you may want to do a clearing if you have had guests over, have had workers in the house, or if you are doing spiritual work there. If you are doing spiritual work as a medium, other type of intuitive reader, or healer, I recommend a space clearing at the end of each day.

There are different techniques that can be used to clear and protect your space of negativity. I generally use white sage followed by holy water. You can find white sage at many spiritual-based book stores or naturalistic or holistic food stores or online retailers. If you do not have white sage or holy water available, you can also use your thoughts to intend and visualize God's white light. Any of these methods will work, as long as the intention is set.

How to Clear and Bless Your Space

Part 1: White Sage

- Open your windows a crack.
- Get out some white sage and an object, such as a large feather or something of substance (like a large greeting card, piece of cardboard), that can be used as a fan.
- Take a small twig of sage, light it, and then put out the flame. You need to burn the sage only a tiny bit, a second or two, working with only the residual smoke to cleanse the space. Always begin at the front door, move in a clockwise direction, and end at the front door.
- State the following *intention* (silently or out loud): "Only spirits who walk in God's white light are welcome here. All negative beings and energies must leave immediately by the power of the I Am [God]."
- As you do this, take the sprig of very mildly smoldering sage and use the feather or other object to fan the smoke to the upper wall or ceiling, along the entire periphery inside the home or other space. In addition, you want to be sure to cover not only the open spaces, but also the top of closets, cupboards, and other closed spaces. Everywhere.
- Be careful. You only need a small sprig of sage and a small amount of smoldering smoke (not a blaze). You want to be care-

So too, you can use these same instructions to clear or cleanse new objects you bring into your space—as well as your own physical person or your loved ones' persons. You may want to do a personal clearing, for example, if you or a loved one is coming home from an environment where there was excessive drinking or drug use. These chemicals make us more

ful not to expose the burning sage to anything flammable and to put out the burning embers completely and store in a safe place when you are finished. You shouldn't be filling the whole place with smoke or burning anything down!

Part 2: Holy Water

- After you clear your space with white sage, you may wish to use holy water to bless and heal.
- Sprinkle the holy water throughout your home or other space (office, school). In each room, sprinkle the holy water in each corner of the room and in the middle of the room.
- As you do this, state the following intention: "Bless this space with love, with love, with love; with light, with light, with light; to heal, to heal, to heal."

Plan B: White Light

- If you do not have sage or holy water available, another option is to state the same two intentions as with the white sage and holy water while visualizing your entire space filling with God's white light.
- Picture the light coming from God, through your heart, and expanding out to all corners of your home or other space (office, school) and beyond.

open, and without the appropriate protection, make us more vulnerable to external energies from both earth and the spirit world. If we are exposed to this type of environment, a personal clearing afterward may be very helpful. In addition, it is important to cleanse any new items that we bring into our space, especially those with a history, such as antique, second-hand, or inherited objects.

PSYCHIC ATTACK. Doing the surround, ground, and shield exercises and regularly cleansing your space and new objects should keep the energy around you and your space clean and positive. However, very rarely, people have reported the presence of a negative energy that arrives unexpectedly or that doesn't want to leave. When a spirit behaves in a way that is menacing, we sometimes call this a *psychic attack*.

This type of "attack" occurs very rarely. If it should happen to you, please use these measures to send this negative energy packing:

- Do not fear. Fear is your worst enemy. Instead, think only of God and God's white light.

   Pray the Lord's Prayer, or Our Father, considered by many to be a universal prayer of protection, or alternatively, use the prayer preferred in your own faith or religion. You can say the prayer out loud or silently to yourself, whichever you are able to do.

   Our Father, who art in heaven, hallowed be Thy name. Thy kingdom come, Thy will be done, on earth as it is in heaven. Give us this day our daily bread and forgive us our trespasses as we forgive those who trespass against us. Lead us not into temptation, but deliver us from evil. For Thine is

> *the kingdom, the power, and the glory forever and
> ever. Amen.*

- As you do this, imagine God's white light and protection springing from within you and radiating throughout your entire home or space.
- Demand the spirit: "No one is allowed in my space unless they are from the light of God."
- Finally, if you do experience a change in your feelings or moods or other symptoms, please state this to the culprit: "Be gone. You are not of me." Say this three times.

Remember: Fear not. The darkness cannot stand in the light. The light always wins.

Ten Seconds a Day

Fortunately, psychic attack is a very rare event and space and personal clearings are needed only periodically. However, this is not the case with our surround, ground, and shield tools. These exercises truly are our daily spiritual defense system, our first steps toward spiritual awareness and healing. And they are easy. But we must to do them each and every day.

Think about it. Would we step out onto a hot beach at midday without putting on the appropriate sunscreen, when we know overexposure to the sun can cause burning and skin cancer? Would we consider going out in the snow without boots or in the rain without an umbrella? And when cold and flu season approaches, would we want to be poorly nourished, dehydrated, and run down so we are even more vulnerable to the virus that's floating around? Or do we want to be proactive about our health and utilize that ounce of prevention?

It's the same with our spiritual health. You can think of these exercises as putting on your sunscreen, taking your vitamins, or wearing your protective gear for the day. You can make the surround, ground, and shield exercises a part of your daily routine, practiced consistently and regularly, at whatever time of the day is best for you. You can also do these exercises multiple times a day when needed. Some people like to do the exercises in the morning, some at bedtime. I recommend you try to do them at the same time each day, as well as using them before you go to work, school, a big event or social outing, or anywhere that you feel you will be in the presence of an overwhelming number of energies or negative, toxic, or unbalanced energies. As we noted, places at increased risk for harboring negative energies include areas where people are drinking excessively or using drugs. In addition, we all know people who have a negative view of life or may vent all of their problems and issues on us. I view these interactions as toxic or toxins—and encounters for which a preventive "surround-ground-shield" may be helpful.

For those who are already suffering, especially those who are empaths, these three exercises alone—practiced regularly and consistently on a daily basis over time—can begin to alleviate or eliminate anxiety, panic attacks, irrational fears, fatigue, and other empath-related symptoms. For some, they will begin to work immediately. For others, it may take a little longer—providing a cumulative effect over time. Including these exercises in our daily routine will also help to maintain our health and balance and reduce or prevent symptoms in the future. For all of us, these exercises can serve as a foundation upon which we can work to heal ourselves and develop our spiritual awareness and gifts.

We really can begin to change our lives, or the lives of our loved ones, in ten seconds a day. And yet with a little more time, energy and, yes, thought, there is so much more.

More to healing. More to you. Are *you* ready for more?

CHAPTER 6

Searching Your Soul: Letting Go of the Hurt

WHEN I THINK BACK TO the time I first took my mother to see a spiritual healer—out of sheer desperation really—I picture those few moments after the session, sitting in the car with her and being amazed at how much lighter she seemed. I didn't yet know whether the healing would have any impact on the widely metastatic cancer that was threatening my mother's life, but she appeared to be so much more at peace. She shared with me that the healer had asked her, "What's eating you up inside?" In fact, there had been something that had been troubling my mother for years, and she felt she had been able to identify this and release it during the healing session. As we know, my mother would go on to live many more years, passing away of other causes at age eighty-four.

I believe dis-ease can be caused by any number of things, from hereditary or genetic predisposition to physical injury to infection, to exposure to environmental toxins (such as those in cigarettes or hazardous chemicals), and the list goes on. I also believe that spiritual, mental, and emotional factors can contribute to the development of symptoms and dis-ease—including anxiety and related symptoms—and that spiritual care can help us to heal and to maintain our health and wellness. An important part of this spiritual care is doing what my mother did: identifying what, if anything, may be eating us up inside. Feelings of hurt, disappointment, sadness, anger, and betrayal are normal and healthy responses in many situations, like the loss of a loved one, a painful relationship, illness, or traumatic event or incident. But from a spiritual perspective, holding on to these negative thoughts and emotions over time can cause a block in our flow of energy, leading to an imbalance in our system and causing a negative impact on our spiritual, mental, emotional, or even physical bodies.

Thank, Bless, and Release

Whatever your hurt is, I cannot tell you that I have experienced or felt the type of pain and suffering you have. I can tell you that it is not your fault when someone else hurts you. I can tell you that you deserve a life of love and peace and happiness and freedom. You deserve the life of your dreams, and you can have it. All people with whom we have a strong interaction in our lives are our teachers. They teach us how to be, and sometimes how not to be. As counterintuitive as it may seem, the way to free yourself from past hurts is to thank God for these teachers and these lessons, and to forgive and release those who have hurt you. We don't have control over those things that happened to us. But we do have control over how we respond to them and whether or not we are going to let them steal the rest of our lives from us. When we hold on to grief, pain, and anger for a prolonged period of time, we are giving our power away and leaving ourselves more vulnerable to other negative thoughts, feelings, and even physical symptoms and dis-ease. All of that hurt and negativity, over time, can make us sick. So you see, forgiveness is for us, not for the persons who hurt us. Forgiving someone doesn't mean that what they did is okay. It means we are taking back our power. It means we are thankful for the lessons we have learned, we release the person or the trauma, loss, or other situation that hurt us, and we let go of the pain we are holding on to—so that we can be free. We thank, bless, and release. This is exactly what Keith and Amy did.

Keith

Keith was thirty-three years old when he came to see me. He was feeling anxious, insecure, and grieving the loss of both of his parents. He had lost his father to cancer when he was just nineteen, and then his mother when he was thirty. He had seen a therapist shortly after his father passed away who helped him cope with the grief over losing his father. He found this to be extremely helpful in moving through that difficult time, but he also noted that the "feeling down" never really went away. With losing his father at such a critical point in his life, he had felt unsure of himself. He was without a role model and mentor, someone to guide him through the following years and chapters of his life. When his mother was diagnosed with cancer and died, his sadness deepened.

Keith's father was an attorney, and Keith was following in his footsteps. He completed his undergraduate studies, struggled through the LSAT exam—three times—went to law school, and ultimately became an attorney himself. When Keith came to see me, he had just become a father for the first time. He was feeling anxious and overwhelmed by the past, and he wanted to learn to enjoy his life so he could be the best husband and father he could be. When Keith and I talked, he was able to identify that he was still grieving the loss of his parents, as well as their guidance and mentorship. He was mourning the fact that his parents wouldn't see him as a father. His children would not know them as grandparents. Keith was also able to recognize that he was still feeling insecure about the fact that he hadn't done as well as he had hoped on the LSAT exam and had received many rejection letters from some of his choice law schools and prospective employers. Even though Keith had long-since graduated from law school and passed the Bar exam, he was still carrying this rejection with him, which was impeding his progress. He just never felt good enough.

Ultimately, I was able to give Keith some tools—including intentions, affirmations, meditations, and visualizations, and other thought and writing exercises—to release what was holding him back so he could embrace his life more fully. I asked Keith to bring in all the rejection letters he had saved and celebrate his release from anxiety and insecurity with a carefully organized shredding ceremony. For Keith, the shredding exercise was a major turning point, a turn toward freedom. He began to change his perspective by focusing less on the pain of his challenges and his parents' passing, and more on being grateful for the time he had with them, for all they gave him and taught him. Keith will always miss his parents, but he has found healing and a new sense of balance and perspective. In addition, he started to use the surround, ground, and shield exercises to protect himself spiritually, and different affirmations to help him gain confidence personally and professionally and move forward in his life. Today, Keith is a successful lawyer, husband, and the father of two sons—and uses the power of gratitude and positive thought to manifest, help others, and live his dream come true.

When we look at the story Keith has shared with us, his pain and anxiety were related to grief and the passing of his loved ones. Many of us have experienced this type of loss and suffering. We are faced with finding a new way to live, to move through the world, without the loved ones who mean so much to us. We may even think if we let go of the sadness, we will let go of the person we love and miss. We think if we love and laugh again, perhaps this means that we love the persons less. But as Keith knows, our loved ones in spirit will always be with us. And we can honor them each and every day by embracing life and the challenges we face with hope and love and joy, which is everything they would want for us.

FOR MANY PEOPLE, it is another type of pain that holds them hostage. Their past hurts are associated with a traumatic event or period of time in their lives. Many were hurt as children, even by a parent or other loved one. Some were neglected or abandoned. Some were part of an abusive relationship or difficult breakup. Some were the victims of assault. Some were falsely accused or treated unfairly or unjustly. Some were made to keep secrets about themselves or others. All of these past hurts can result in feelings of anger, sadness, fear, mistrust, guilt, shame, worthlessness, and insecurity.

Amy

Like Keith, Amy suffered with anxiety, panic, and feelings of depression. But Amy's pain came from another place. When Amy first e-mailed me about her severe anxiety and her experiences with seeing and receiving messages from the spirit world, I was so moved by her message that I called her immediately after reading it. Amy was seven months pregnant at the time, was experiencing extreme anxiety and panic attacks, and her father had been urging her to contact me for help. On the phone, she explained that she had been "seeing dead people" since she was three years old. As a child, she was afraid to tell anyone about these experiences, because she was raised in a very religious setting and wasn't sure this type of thing would be considered "of God." So she hid and suppressed her gifts as best as she could and tried to manage her feelings of anxiety and depression. Now thirty-three years old, the visions and messages from spirit were still coming and she thought she just might be crazy.

I assured Amy that she was not crazy or evil, that she was an empath and was spiritually gifted. After learning to apply the surround, ground, and shield exercises, Amy was able to reduce her anxiety and panic attacks significantly. I also advised her that she was in control of her interactions with spirit, and that she needed to set Do Not Disturb time periods, when they were not to communicate with her, and this helped as well. However, a few days after she gave birth to her new baby, Amy awoke in the night in a panic, seeing and hearing spirits. She called me at about 1:00 a.m. I was able to help her breathe through the panic attack and did a healing on her by phone. In talking with Amy further, we were able to determine that her feelings of anxiety and depression resulted not only from her being an empath and repressing strong spiritual gifts, but also from years of physical, sexual, and emotional abuse in her childhood. She didn't trust people. She didn't have a sense of personal boundaries. Emotionally, she didn't know where she ended and others started. As part of Amy's healing, she had to work on taking care of herself, on setting and trusting her boundaries with both human and spiritual beings, on trusting her own feelings and perceptions, and on letting go of the pain that was keeping her prisoner.

Ultimately, Amy chose to forgive those who had hurt her, so that she could move forward into wholeness and happiness, for herself and her children. Today, Amy works as a spiritual medium and healer. Her children are also gifted—and they are proud of it.

———

Now, just as we need to forgive those who have hurt us, we must also forgive ourselves for the hurts we have caused. We have all made mistakes. We have all missed opportunities. We have all said or done something hurtful, or not said or not done what we should have, at different points in our lives. But we are not our mistakes and our shortcomings. We can choose to believe the lie that we are the sum of our failures and accomplishments, or we can believe the truth that we are much, much more.

When possible, it's important to express an apology and make amends to those we have hurt, so that we can assist in their healing process. If it isn't possible or won't be helpful to apologize in person—for example, perhaps the injured party is deceased or maybe an apology would cause even more hurt and disruption for the person—then we can do so by thought, sending our apology, healing, and love. Most importantly, we need to learn from our mistakes so that we continue to become the kinder, gentler, more loving souls we are meant to be. We can honor the people who have been our teachers, thank the Universe for our lessons, and forgive others and ourselves. We choose to love ourselves, so we can move forward in love and service to others.

Whether we are forgiving ourselves or others, there are a few tools that can be effective in facilitating this process. Two of these include a forgiveness meditation, the other a forgiveness letter. Before you begin this or any meditation, please be sure to do your surround, ground, and shield exercises (chapter 5).

Learning to Forgive Through Meditation

This meditation is designed to help you release negative programs that you have accumulated throughout your lifetime, and to forgive those who had a part in creating them. Patterns of guilt, fear, shame, anger and judgment, as well as issues that have

affected your self-esteem. Issues that have been created, or been contributed to by interactions with your
parents, siblings, teachers, and anyone else that may
have had a negative effect on you throughout your
childhood and adult life

- ⟶ I would like you to sit quietly now, in a comfortable position, close your eyes, and begin by
  breathing in through your nose to the count of
  four...holding it for four...and blowing it out
  your mouth for four.
- ⟶ And again, all the way into your abdomen...
  hold it...and blow it all the way out your mouth.
- ⟶ Now begin to imagine or feel your energy field
  expanding as you breathe, until it fills the entire room.
- ⟶ You are already beginning to feel lighter and
  lighter as your energy pushes against the ceiling.
- ⟶ Continue to expand until you have left the
  room and find yourself ascending all the way
  out of the room where you began.
- ⟶ You are so far above now that you can see or
  imagine the houses and buildings far below
  you. The streets and the cars have become
  smaller as your energy continues to rise.
- ⟶ Now imagine yourself all the way out in space.
  Feel how much lighter your energy is now.
- ⟶ Send thoughts of love and light to everyone and
  everything on the planet.
- ⟶ Love and light are positive thought forms that
  are powerful enough to change the world in
  which you live. When you transmit love and light
  from your heart to others, it circles right back to

you. You begin to feel a sense of peace as you realize that we are all part of the same energy.

→ A beautiful tunnel of rainbow lights has suddenly opened before you. Your spirit guide
awaits you inside and he or she has been with
you since before you were born to this earth.
Step into the tunnel and feel the unconditional
love that your guide has for you.

→ Your guide is going to accompany you to a
place where all of the people that you have had
important interactions with are lined up.

→ When you reach them you will be returning to
them all of the old programs that were created
by them and taken on by you. They were never
yours to hold in the first place. If you have nothing to return to someone, just send them love.

→ Begin with your parents and your siblings, one
by one, return all of the shame, the guilt, the
fears, the anxieties, the judgments, and the expectations that were placed upon you by your
family members. Give them back with love, no
accusations or resentments. You are simply returning them to where they belong.

→ Now, standing in front of you is any partner or
spouse that you have had in this lifetime, as
well as any in-laws. Return any negative emotions that had been placed upon you, always
with love.

→ You are beginning to feel lighter every time
you release the negative programming and
thought forms.

→ Now, in front of you stand any children or
friends that you may have difficulties with.

> Give them their programs back, one at a time, with love.

→ Now, perhaps an employer or co-worker with whom you may have unresolved issues.

→ You have now released all negativity from your energy field and you feel so much lighter, it is such an uplifting feeling.

→ I would like you now to thank them all and bless them for all of the lessons they have taught you in this life. Some have taught you what to do and others have taught you what never to do. Some may have given you courage, others strength, perhaps even the gift of life or the gift of survival. They are the foundation of your personality. Embrace this foundation!

→ It is time now to release all of your own negative programming that you have placed upon yourself. Release any negative thoughts with love and only take with you the positive lessons that you have learned throughout this life.

→ You find yourself letting out a huge sigh of relief as you recognize that the secret to life has always been to love yourself.

→ Now imagine your guide escorting you back through the rainbow tunnel in preparation for your return. Thank your guide for all of the time spent helping you and all the love that has been directed toward you each and every day.

→ Step outside of the tunnel and find yourself, once again, out in the Universe, floating closer and closer to the earth…as your energy field begins to slowly contract.

➤ Imagine now or feel yourself above the town and beginning the descent into the room where you began your journey of forgiveness...knowing you are better for having done this.

➤ And simply now, by closing your hands into a fist, and slowly, gently, opening your eyes, you come back into the space where you began.*

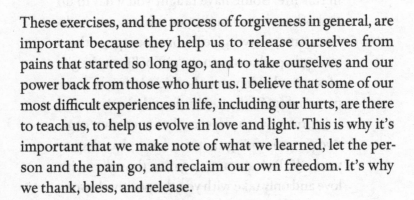

These exercises, and the process of forgiveness in general, are important because they help us to release ourselves from pains that started so long ago, and to take ourselves and our power back from those who hurt us. I believe that some of our most difficult experiences in life, including our hurts, are there to teach us, to help us evolve in love and light. This is why it's important that we make note of what we learned, let the person and the pain go, and reclaim our own freedom. It's why we thank, bless, and release.

Finding Support

Finally, recalling past hurts, traumas, and loss can be difficult and confusing, and we should not go through this process alone. As you seek to identify these issues and let them go in order to heal, I recommend reaching out to trusted family and friends. Some people find support groups extremely helpful.

---

* This meditation can be done as often as needed. You can also find this guided meditation on "Guided Meditations with Pat Longo" on iTunes, Amazon, and other digital platforms.

The Forgiveness Letter

This exercise is exactly what it sounds like: a letter of forgiveness to each person who has hurt us. The intention of this letter is not to hurt the "recipient" or others, but to take our power back. This letter should be handwritten, not saved electronically.

- In this letter, I would like you to document what the person did that hurt you, how it made you feel, and how it affected you.
- Make sure to get everything—all the pain, all the suffering—down in the letter.
- You may want to add what you have learned from this experience—and thank the person that, by his or her actions, has taught you what NOT to say or do, how NOT to be. If you do not feel comfortable thanking the person, you can instead say "I thank God for the lessons I've learned through this experience" and indicate what they are. Or you can write a separate letter to God, to thank, bless, and release this person, the hurt, and the situation.
- In your letter, state that you are releasing the person who hurt you and the hurt itself, you are blessing the situation, and you are taking your power back.
- At the end of the letter, state very simply, "I thank you, I bless you, and I release you."
- **This is very important**: While and after you write this letter, do NOT read the letter. Do NOT send the letter. Do NOT share the letter. Do NOT leave the letter where others may see it. Destroy the letter immediately. The point of the letter is to use thoughts and words to get all the hurt out and release it. To read the letter would be to take it right back in. Once the letter is finished, it can be shredded, burned, or otherwise destroyed in a responsible and safe manner.

You may also want to work with a professional psychologist, psychotherapist, or counselor. A trusted clergy member or spiritual counselor may also be able to provide useful guidance and support. It is important to find the therapist or counselor who is right for you—and a referral from your physician or a friend may be helpful. As Keith has shared, his therapist was instrumental in helping him adjust to living with the loss of his father at a very sensitive time in his life. And as we know, Keith is now living and appreciating a life filled with happiness and love.

Whatever your suffering may be—anxiety, fear, worry, depression, sadness, anger, shame, feelings of worthlessness or hopelessness—I ask you to make the commitment to search your heart and soul to identify any past hurts that may be contributing to your pain and to let them go.

Choose you, and you can break out of the prison of the past. Choose you, and you can be free. Free to heal. Free to have the life and love that is your soul's destiny. Free to raise even higher and shine even brighter.

CHAPTER 7

Making Spirits
Bright...and Light

A S WE CONTINUE TO HEAL ourselves, it's important to remember why we are here. Each of us has undertaken this
human journey with our own agreement with God, our own
quest for spiritual growth and evolvement, our own unique
soul's purpose or calling on our life. To answer this calling, we
must begin with loving ourselves—and with raising our own
energetic vibration to that of a consciousness of love. We are
here to raise ourselves and each other up.

If the entire Universe is made of energy, moving at different vibrations or frequencies, and we too are energy, then we
are constantly using, projecting, and drawing to us energy, either for positive or negative. On the path to spiritual
enlightenment, we are learning to raise our energetic vibration to that of God, to that of love. God and love in all of its
many forms—compassion, gratitude, generosity, goodness,
kindness, contentment, forgiveness, mercy, grace, joy—carry

the highest vibration of energy. Thus, positive thoughts, feelings, and states of being such as these can help us to raise our vibration. Negative thoughts and feelings—such as hatred, judgment, anger, jealousy, spite, sadness, guilt, shame, and blame—can carry energy of a lower vibration. I believe that using our thoughts to raise our vibration can help to keep us in a state of energy balance and flow. This balanced state is one that can best foster an environment of healing, health, and wholeness over time—and help us to manifest our best lives and facilitate the fulfillment of our soul's purpose. I also believe that holding on to negative thoughts can make us more vulnerable to imbalance and dis-ease (including symptoms such as anxiety), and thus can slow or stop us from walking into our full destiny. Indeed, it is in working toward this state of high vibration and balance that we can best open to our whole selves—including to the spiritual gifts that are ours to discover, accept, and develop in a responsible, balanced way.

We all know what it feels like to be lifted in heart and spirit by a joyful or happy moment. And we know how it feels when a person with a warm smile or wonderful laugh enters our space. These positive thoughts and emotions can raise us right up. They can transform the room. Happiness is a wonderful place to be. It's also important to know that there are other ways to raise our vibration, other ways to inspire and to love ourselves and others, and not all of them come with a happy face all of the time. In fact, some of them can come in our most challenging moments.

I believe that negative thoughts and feelings can make us more vulnerable to dis-ease. And dis-ease can make us more vulnerable to negativity. However, this does not mean people who are experiencing loss, trauma, sadness, or dis-ease necessarily have a low vibration or are negative. By design, we all face challenges in our lives in order to learn and grow spiritually. It is how we respond to these challenges that will determine whether we move forward in a positive or negative way, with a higher or lower vibration.

For example, we have seen individuals in our own lives and in the news who have experienced trauma and loss and have responded by doing all they could to bring something positive from a negative situation. We know people who have been diagnosed with cancer, or lost a loved one to cancer, and in their sorrow have reached out to raise awareness and research funds for others who may be faced with this diagnosis. We have seen those born with a disability or debilitating disease use their lives to inspire others. We saw Christopher and Dana Reeve rally after a tragic accident to help advance research in spinal cord injury. Michael J. Fox turned his experience with Parkinson's into an effort to increase awareness and research around this dis-ease. Katie Couric took the tragic death of her husband from colon cancer and used it to help save lives through increasing awareness to promote screening and prevention and raising funds for research. John Walsh, who lost a child to violence, dedicated his life to fighting crime and helping others find their missing children. Many of the families and friends who have lost loved ones, including children, in mass shootings, while grief-stricken and heartbroken, have chosen to try to use their loss as a teachable moment to create meaningful change in hearts and minds. There are many more people, public and private, who are turning devastating circumstances into hope and inspiration for others. I believe people like these, though they were or are experiencing difficult times and emotions, have responded in a way that raises their vibration and, indeed, raises us all. Those moving through hurtful, challenging situations may not feel or look joyful and happy all of the time. None of us does. But they are extending themselves in love, in compassion, and often in gratitude for the time they were able to share with the loved one they lost. So while I believe living in or hanging on to negativity lowers our vibration and can make us sick, it's important to know that being sick or feeling grief or sadness or pain in and of itself does not mean we have a low vibration. It's in how we respond. Indeed, responding to a challenge or hurt can bring us to our greatest learning and our highest love.

To maintain our healing and health and to achieve the spiritual growth we desire, we want to set our intention to work consciously every day to raise our vibration. We can do this using the power of thought to enhance our connection with spirit, protect our energy, replace the negative with the positive, and love ourselves and others.

Connecting with Spirit

To raise our vibration, we want to live from a perspective of spiritual awareness, in connection and communication with our higher selves, our spirit guides, and God. To help develop and maintain this spiritual connection, a few simple measures may be helpful.

First, prayer is a simple form of connecting with and talking to God. We may use prayer to thank God, to ask Him for guidance or assistance for ourselves and others, even to say hello. We can use prayers that originate from our own spiritual or religious backgrounds or practices, or we can simply speak to God in our own thoughts and words. If you don't use the term "God," then use whatever name you use to refer to the higher power, the source or higher consciousness of goodness. When in prayer, it's important to be positive and to pray with the intention for the highest good of all. We don't want to ask for anything negative and we don't want to ask in a way that limits us. Sometimes we think we know what's best for us or others, but God has an even bigger, better something planned. On this same note, it's important that we put gratitude in our prayers. I send my own prayers with a "thank you" rather than a "please."

Second, meditation is a powerful way to connect with our higher self, spirit guides, and God. I recommend meditating with this intention at least three times per week for five, ten, or fifteen minutes at a time. To do this type of meditation, we can use thought to help take us to a level of consciousness where our mind becomes free of thought and chatter and we are simply present with ourselves and God. We are, in essence, "listening" to God. We can also use this method to listen to our spirit guides and others in the spiritual realm.

There are many ways to use thought to achieve this state of meditation. One way is to focus on something specific, like our breathing. Another way is to use our imagination, to envision a story or place that will serve as a bridge to the meditative state. You can do this independently or with a guided meditation. The Creating Your Sacred Space Meditation is included here to get you started. Please be sure to do your ten-second surround, ground, and shield exercises before starting the meditation.

Creating Your Sacred Space Meditation

This meditation is designed to help you to create a sacred space for yourself.

⤳ I would like you to begin by sitting in a comfortable space or perhaps lying down.

- ⇀ Closing your eyes now, breathe in through your nose to the count of 4 and slowly blow it out your mouth.
- ⇀ Repeating the breath again, all the way in and all the way out.
- ⇀ Now, imagine yourself standing at the edge of a pine-needle forest.
- ⇀ The path is very inviting.
- ⇀ Step onto the path and feel the warmth of the sun on your face as it filters through the treetops.
- ⇀ There are wild flowers scattered about.
- ⇀ The birds are chirping.
- ⇀ And small animals are scurrying about from tree to tree.
- ⇀ It is so peaceful and tranquil as you walk upon the path.
- ⇀ At the end of the path, you reach a clearing and find a magnificent meadow.
- ⇀ The grass moving ever so gently in the breeze.
- ⇀ There is a small brook off to the side, and you can hear the sounds of the stream as it moves over the rocks.
- ⇀ Majestic trees surround the edge of the meadow, like mighty protectors.
- ⇀ This is your sacred space. No one can enter unless invited by you.
- ⇀ Find a place to rest, perhaps at the base of a tree or on a large rock at the edge of the brook or on the soft green grass of the meadow.
- ⇀ Feel the safety and tranquility of your sacred space and know that you can come here at will, simply by thought, any time you feel the need for solace or reflection.

- ⇀ And know that you are one with your maker.
- ⇀ And simply now, by closing your hands into a fist, and opening your eyes, come back to the space where you began, knowing that you are better for having done this.*

While meditating, if your to-do list, the laundry that needs to be done, the appointment you have to make, or other thoughts or worries pop into your mind, this is okay. Just allow it, put these thoughts in a bubble, and let them float away. It's also okay if you experience thoughts or feelings of anxiety or worry while meditating. Just breathe, let them come, and let them go. If you find yourself not listening to the exact words, drifting off into your own spiritual experience, that's fine too. This means that your imagination is serving as the bridge to your own meditative, spiritual state. As you begin to meditate regularly, the process of reaching and maintaining a meditative state will become easier and you may wish to increase gradually the length of time you spend with these exercises. The purpose is simply for you to develop the ability to connect with your spiritual self during these short sessions. You do not need to achieve any type of milestone or experience; you just need to continue doing the meditations regularly and the desired effect will develop over time, even if you are not feeling this in the beginning. Just keep setting the time aside and doing the exercises, and you will do just fine.

---

* This meditation can be done as often as you wish. You can also find this guided meditation on my YouTube channel at www.youtube.com/user/thepat longochannel.

Third, many of us find that visiting sacred places helps to facilitate our spiritual connection. Often, we find God in nature. Spending time strolling in the park, walking on the beach, viewing a sunset, fishing on your favorite river bank, or even sitting quietly with the birds in the backyard may help you to connect with the Divine and also with the earth. And finally, if you have a belief system that lends itself to a spiritual or religious practice, sharing and celebrating God in prayer, song, and service with others who have similar beliefs can be helpful to maintaining your spiritual connection. Attending church, temple, mosque, or other group services and activities can bring a sense of shared community, inspiration, and love. Where two or more are gathered in God's name…good things can happen.

Protecting and Grounding

An important next step in keeping our vibration high is protecting ourselves from external energies that may be negative, toxic, or unbalanced. We want to maintain positive thoughts and emotions and prevent this negative energy, either from earth or the spirit world, from influencing us. To ensure we are protected spiritually, we need to remember to use our spiritual defense system—our surround, ground, and shield exercises (visit chapter 5)—each and every day.

It also bears repeating: Grounding is as important as—or even more important than—anything else related to raising our vibration. Remember, we are spiritual beings having a human experience. We are essentially both heaven and earth. As we work to raise our vibration, our spiritual connection becomes stronger and we rise higher. In terms of a visual metaphor, if we imagine our earthly energy as an electric fan with the blades still, then our spiritual energy, at a higher vibration, would appear as that same fan with the blades turning so rapidly that they appear as one big blur. Because we must maintain this high vibration while functioning on earth, we must make sure our spiritual-mental-emotional-physical bodies are in a state of balance. We can do this by balancing our efforts to raise our spiritual energy with grounding into the earth's energy. There are many people who are highly spiritually connected, who are exceptionally gifted or sensitive, whose vibration is very high. Yet, many don't know that they need to ground themselves as well as connect spiritually. For this reason, they are out of balance. These people can appear as though they are living in another dimension. They may seem to be "flighty," "out of it," "always in their head," or otherwise disconnected. For those of us living on earth, grounding is absolutely essential.

Eliminating the Negative, Accentuating the Positive

Our thoughts are our most powerful tools to raise our vibration and realize more fully our Divine selves on earth. Our thoughts become things, and once we focus on them or speak them or write them, they *are* things. To raise our vibrations and create the lives we want, we need to eliminate negativity within ourselves and in our surroundings. In doing this, we make even more room for the positive!

HAVE FAITH, NOT FEAR. My first rule of thought is *have faith, not fear*. Just as darkness cannot stand in the light, fear cannot exist in the presence of faith. Have faith in God and in who you are and where you are from. If you experience fear, use your thoughts to say the Lord's Prayer (Our Father) (or the preferred prayer of your faith), call upon God, or simply visualize God's white light pouring into you and the space around you. Franklin Delano Roosevelt was right: "The only thing we have to fear is fear itself." Just kick it to the curb.

BLESS AND RELEASE. As Keith and Amy showed us, a big part of healing comes with identifying the source of our pain and suffering (chapter 6). Holding on to negative thoughts and experiences can lower our vibration. Releasing these deep hurts can help us to heal and to raise our vibration. When you let go of your old hurt, pain, anger, and toxic thoughts and feelings, you will not only eliminate this negative hold on your life, but you will create a space for all of the wonderful, positive things that are coming your way.

THANK YOU, THANK YOU, THANK YOU. I believe gratitude may be the quickest, easiest way to take our energy from the basement to the ceiling. Indeed, gratitude is a transformational force that can change our lives and change the world. You can integrate gratitude into your life in simple, easy ways. One way is the use of a gratitude journal, making a list of three to five things you are grateful for each day.

Another way is in our intentions and prayers. When you wish to intend or pray for something, you can use the phrase *thank you* instead of *please*. For example, don't pray, "Please help me to find a job soon." Instead pray, "Thank you for sending me the job that is right for me." (We should still say please when asking for the mashed potatoes at the dinner table.)

And of course, we should say thank you, thank you, thank you as much as possible—to all those who help and support and love us in this life. We are all on this journey together and none of us is going to do it alone. Sometimes, "thank you" can be the difference between someone feeling heartbroken and feeling validated, loved, and full of heart.

THOUGHTS AND WORDS. We all have a kind of "audiotape" that plays in our minds, and we want to make it a positive one. It is important to be mindful of the thoughts you think and the words you choose to speak, sign, or write. Remember, you are creating your life every moment of every day. And once you give voice to your thoughts, they *are* things. There are some simple tips you can use to help ensure that you are thinking and speaking positively, at the highest possible vibration.

First, it's important to set your intention, both in advance and in the moment, to be mindful of your thoughts and words and to work each day to use them for the highest good.

Second, I recommend you do this, not by trying to stop the negative thoughts from coming. This will only give them more focus and energy. Rather, you want to work proactively to think positively and replace any negative thoughts that do occur with positive thoughts.

You can begin to do this by preparing in advance a list of positive affirmations that you will say to yourself several times a day, out loud or silently. These affirmations will also serve as tools at-the-ready, should you have negative thoughts that need replacement with the positive. Examples of such positive affirmations are listed here:

- *I am.*
- *I am thankful for . . .*
- *I am peace.*
- *I am love.*
- *I am cancer-free.*
- *I am healthy and balanced in spirit, mind, heart, and body.*

- *I have a strong and healthy immune system and am getting better every day.*
- *I move through life with flexibility and ease.*
- *I receive and give love freely.*
- *The Universe is conspiring in my favor.*
- *I choose to forgive and to take back my life.*
- *I choose joy.*
- *I choose love.*

You can use any of these or create your own affirmations, tailoring them to your own situation. It's okay if you do not see or feel these thoughts and words. You just have to intend them.

Similarly, it's important to become more aware of other words that can be frequently thought or spoken mindlessly. Much like using the words "thank you" instead of "please" in prayer and affirmation, you also need to be careful how you use your words in day-to-day life. To start, *I am* may be the two most powerful words in the history of language. Whatever you place after *I am* is what you are becoming. For example:

- Instead of "I am feeling anxious" or "I am a nervous wreck," breathe and state "I am feeling more and more calm" or "My mind is like a crystal-clear lake with no ripples, becoming more and more calm."
- Instead of "I am not feeling well," say "I am feeling better all the time." In fact, James Brown may not know it, but he is one of my biggest cheerleaders in helping me to raise my vibration and manifest health and wellness in my life. When I occasionally wake up feeling a little under the weather, I launch straight into one of his greatest hits: "I Feel Good." And yes, I sing it out loud! And yes, I admit I may dance a little too.

- Don't say "I am a diabetic" or "I am a paraplegic" or "I am an epileptic" or "I am autistic" or "I am a cancer patient." Really? Is that who you are? I don't think so. Say instead, "I was diagnosed with diabetes" or "I was diagnosed with a spinal cord injury" (or epilepsy or autism or cancer). You may have been diagnosed with a dis-ease, you may be fighting it, you may be learning or teaching lessons through the experience of it, you may be beating it, you may be healing from it—but you are not a dis-ease. You may be using a wheelchair as transportation, but you are not a wheelchair or the condition that has made the wheelchair necessary. A dis-ease does not own or define you. A wheelchair does not own or define you. It is not who you are.

- Instead of saying "I am flat broke," say something like "I have more than enough abundance to live a comfortable life," "There is no limit to the blessings and abundance of God," or "I thank God for His blessings and abundance in my life."

- Similarly, it's important to be careful with other damaging words and phrases that we sometimes use mindlessly. Phrases such as "you're killing me," "my back is killing me," "this is never going to work," or "I'll never pass this test." We don't want these thoughts and words going out into the Universe. I recommend you replace these words in your vocabulary with positive intentions and affirmations. Say instead: "My back is feeling better every day" and "Thank you that this [situation] is working for the highest good of all."

Finally, if you think or say something negative by mistake, you can take it back! You can simply say the words (when in public, silently is usually best): "Cancel, cancel." This is how you make your intention known to the Universe, putting a halt to any inadvertent negativity.

Using these techniques, you will find that, over time, your positive thoughts and words will grow more prevalent and your negative thoughts will dissipate.

MEDIA AND ENTERTAINMENT. Everything we put into ourselves changes us. Just as we need to protect ourselves spiritually with the surround, ground, and shield exercises, so too we need to protect ourselves from other toxins. This includes exposure to violent, base, or otherwise negative media and entertainment, whether it's television, movies, radio, social media, video games, or literature. It's important for you to limit this exposure as much as possible and find forms of entertainment and enjoyment that inspire you.

ALCOHOL AND DRUG USE. The overuse of alcohol or use of mood-altering drugs has a negative impact on our systems, both immediately and in the long term. Spiritually, these chemicals both lower our vibration and make us more open to surrounding energies. In addition to the mental and physical effects we feel, an overuse of alcohol or use of these drugs leaves us extremely vulnerable to negative spiritual energies. For many people, alcohol in moderation can be fine. If you are planning to enjoy a glass of wine at a social event or with dinner, I recommend that you simply complete the ten-second surround, ground, and shield exercises—and add the exercise to imagine a zipper, zipping up and closing your seven main chakras for extra protection—just before the first sip.

TOXIC FRIENDS. It is important to choose our friends wisely. We all have difficult or challenging times in life when we need our family and friends to listen, to offer comfort, and to hold us up and support us through. But if you have friends who are consistently taking, abusing, having a negative or fatalistic attitude, or leaving you feeling drained, you may want to limit your time with them or find more positive friends. Oftentimes, this process happens quite naturally on its own. As you raise your vibration higher, you will see friends who have a more negative outlook phase out of your life because they are no longer getting what they want from the relationship. Ultimately, you need to surround yourself with people who love and support you and who are dedicated to a higher good.

Similarly, if there are individuals with whom you are experiencing challenges, it's important to take the "high road." This can happen with family, friends, colleagues, or even people online or on social media. For any of these situations, I recommend using the intention to send pink light to these individuals, whenever a difficulty occurs:

> *Simply think of the person and imagine sending a beam of pink light from your heart to the other person's heart. The pink light represents love. As you are imagining this, you can visualize it in your mind's eye. But if you can't visualize it, it's okay. You don't have to see or feel anything with this exercise. You just have to intend it.*

Remember, *thoughts become things*. Taking this higher road, so to speak, will help you, help the person to whom you are sending the light, aid in resolving the situation for the highest good, and send more love out to the Universe. It's a win-win-win-win.

GOOD-VIBRATIONS LIBRARY. One of the best ways to raise our vibration is to think about and surround ourselves with the people, things, and activities that we love. If we are having a bad day—feeling sad or upset—merely thinking of the people and things that bring us love, laughter, and joy can fill our hearts and raise our vibration. I recommend that you build in advance a library of joyful, inspiring thoughts, memories, or moments to have at-the-ready, so that when you need them, you can put them right to work.

Your own good-vibrations library may include items such as these:

- **LOVE.** Create a list of love-ly moments in your life. These are moments in which people have extended themselves in kindness to you, or special moments you have shared with those you love. Let the love shine a light in your heart and radiate out through your whole being.
- **GRATITUDE.** I think of gratitude as a highly transformational form of love. Make a list or think of people or things for which you are grateful. Let gratitude lift you up.
- **PRIDE.** Make another list! This one should include qualities, moments, or accomplishments of which you are proud. This is not meant in a boastful or egocentric way, but is simply a method of reminding yourself of who you are, where you come from, and the good that you have done—and can do.
- **LAUGHTER.** Think of a person, animal, story, memory, or even comedian that makes you smile or laugh.
- **MUSIC.** Think of or listen to a favorite song that makes you feel joyful and happy.
- **BEAUTY.** Think of, read, or visit something that feeds your soul with beauty and grace. Some may find beauty in a favorite poem, a work of art or art mu-

seum, theater, dance performance, or places or things in nature (a park, beach, mountain range, sunset, ocean, trees, wild animals).

- **PHOTOS OR VIDEOS.** Do you have photos or videos that make you smile or warm your heart? Perhaps a video of something a small child said or did, a pet enjoying the park, or a celebratory event? Keep them handy and use them to lift you up when you need it.
- **PEOPLE WHO RAISE US UP.** There are people who have a way of lifting other people up. Whoever this is in your life—whether a parent, sibling, aunt or uncle, friend, or even clergy member—reach out to them and let them help you gain perspective and see the good in a challenging situation.

Loving Yourself

When we talk about our journey to heal and to raise our vibration to that of love, it's so important to remember that this includes love of the self. We cannot heal and we cannot love God and others to our full potential if we do not love ourselves. For many of us, this is the most difficult part of our journey and our lessons here on earth. Some of us have simply lost ourselves in the hustle and bustle of day-to-day living. Others feel emotional pain or shame over hurtful things that have been said or done to us. People have told us that our voices were not worth hearing, that our thoughts and feelings did not matter, that we were not important. Some of us have been told that there was something wrong with us or some part of us. We play these voices over and over again in our minds and feel these feelings, day in and day out, in our hearts.

And little by little, we start hiding parts of ourselves away, walling off our hearts, living in fragments. And one day, we look around and we don't know where we went. Even more heartbreaking to me is that this lack of self-esteem and self-worth prevents us from embracing our whole selves and fully realizing our soul's purpose. The truth is, these things that we were told were lies, fed to us by people who themselves were broken and in need of healing.

So if you've never had anyone tell you before, let me tell you now. You are here. You matter. You are beautiful. You are loved. You have the entire Universe and all of its vast wonder and possibility and potential within you. Indeed, the very presence of God resides within you.

If you are lacking in self-esteem or self-worth, feeling like you're lost, aren't enough, or just don't know who you are anymore, it's important that you make a conscious choice to stop believing the lies and to commit to renewing your sense of self-love. There are several exercises I recommend to help people begin to open their hearts and find their way back to loving themselves. One is the Learning to Forgive Through Meditation exercise (chapter 6), which is helpful for facilitating forgiveness of the self and letting go of past issues that are

Self-Love Affirmation

- Please go into a room with a mirror where you can be alone.
- Look at yourself in the mirror.
- Say to yourself in the mirror, "I love you."
- Please repeat this exercise twice (or more) per day, preferably as you begin and end your day, every day.

keeping us from loving and accepting ourselves. Two other exercises, included here, are focused directly on love of self. Will you give them a try with me?

Loving Yourself Meditation

This meditation is designed to help you open to and love your whole self. I would like you to begin by sitting in a comfortable space or perhaps lying down, and closing your eyes.

- → As you relax in the rhythm of your breath, envision your special place or sanctuary. This is your place in your mind's eye where you feel safe, secure, and at peace. It may be a garden or waterfall or perhaps a meadow.
- → Sit or lie down in your special place and begin to feel even more relaxed and at one with all of life.
- → Turn your attention to the area around your heart.
- → This is the center of unconditional love.
- → See or feel this area being filled by a beautiful pink light of love.
- → Any tightness around this area is now being alleviated.
- → The healing light of love is clearing all the old hurts and pains that have been stored in your heart.
- → Continue to let this beautiful pink light mend and repair feelings of hurt.
- → As it does, visualize or imagine the area around your heart expanding with love and compassion.

- ⇀ Let this center fill with as much healing energy as you can possibly imagine.
- ⇀ I'd like you now to encircle yourself with this wonderful pink healing light of love.
- ⇀ Let this energy absorb all your doubts and fears so that you feel clear and free of them.
- ⇀ Allow this light to fill your entire being with unconditional love.
- ⇀ No matter what you have said or done to yourself in the past, this pink light absorbs it until it is gone.
- ⇀ Any time you need to love who you are, you can return to your sanctuary and use this amazing pink healing light to expand your heart center.
- ⇀ Now go about your day, feeling love and giving love.
- ⇀ And simply now, by closing your hands into a fist, and opening your eyes, come back to the space where you began, knowing that you are better for having done this.*

While these two exercises are technically very quick and easy, for many people, they are emotionally and spiritually the most challenging they will do. Even if you don't feel the words, even if it is uncomfortable at first, please do these exercises every day. Over time, your heart will begin to feel and come alive to this expression of love and compassion.

---

* This meditation can be done daily. You can also find this guided meditation on my YouTube channel at www.youtube.com/user/thepatlongochannel.

Remember also that loving yourself, means loving your whole self, including your intuition and related spiritual gifts. I cannot tell you the incredible number of people I have met who had been hiding or suppressing their spiritual gifts simply because they had been told that they were ill, crazy, or even evil. These were frequently individuals who had particularly strong gifts, the emergence and expression of which resulted in fear or ridicule.

For those of you who are hiding or not embracing your spiritual gifts out of fear or shame, I will just come right out and say it: It's okay to recognize and embrace your intuition. It's okay to have psychic, mediumship, and spiritual healing abilities. These are beautiful gifts that God has given to you to develop and share, as part of your life's purpose.

A particularly sad thing for me is that people often are told by those claiming to be spiritual or religious that these gifts are not from God, but from evil. I remember my own mother asking me how I knew that my gift of healing was from God and not from something sinister. This was after her own life had been saved by a spiritual healer, after being told by her doctor that she would not live much more than a year due to widely metastatic breast cancer. And still today, so many people come to me, fearful of their gifts. I can recall one client calling, terribly distressed when a friend found out that she had the gift of mediumship. This friend referred her to passages in the Bible that she believed indicated the evil nature of this gift.

I told my mother that I am using the abilities that God gave me to help others. I told her I am not hurting people, I am doing my best to help people. How could that be evil? I told her I work for God and only God—and I feel a calling to use the gifts that God has given me. I believe we all need to accept and love ourselves and all that God has made us to be. And when we learn to love and raise ourselves up, we will have all the more love to offer to others.

Helping Others

What better way to raise our vibration, to call into being our brightest and lightest Divine selves, than to love and be of service to others? Whether it's volunteering at a hospital, church, homeless shelter, nursing home, or reaching out to a friend who is ill or neighbor who is homebound, helping someone else is a sure way to lift them up, lift ourselves up, and send love and light into the world.

So now you have your homework. These are the tools and information you will need to help you stay spiritually connected, protected, grounded, balanced, and light today and every day after. Our next stop is energy healing. Come with me... and you'll see.

CHAPTER 8

The Energy Healing

*H*EALING, IN MY EXPERIENCE, IS the process of bringing one's whole self into balance, in love and light, and opening the pathway for one to be fully realized in all God meant him or her to be.

In our partnership of healing so far, we have covered almost all of the steps I provide in my sessions to help you heal and to maintain a protected, grounded, balanced state of being in spirit-mind-heart-body. The last step I provide is the one for which many people seek out a spiritual healer in the first place, that of the energy healing. The practice of energy healing can come in many different forms, and may be referred to by many different names, including spiritual healing, natural energy healing, hands-on healing, faith healing, and others. Different healers may practice different forms and methods of energy healing. I call myself a spiritual healer or natural energy healer, and the method I use to facilitate an energy healing is one that has evolved over time, based upon my own intuition and inner guidance and the lessons I have learned along the way.

Love, Light, and Intention

In my practice, I facilitate an energy healing using three key elements: love, light, and intention. For ages, light has been a symbol of goodness, truth, love, God. In the case of spiritual healing, it is not only a symbol, but a powerful reality. I use my intention to become a vessel to connect with the love, light, and healing energy of God, or Universal Life Force energy, to bring healing through myself and into the recipient for the highest good of the recipient and all concerned. In doing so, I am serving as a channel for this love, light, and healing energy to ground and balance the individual's energy—clearing and balancing the chakras and the spiritual, mental, emotional, and physical bodies, removing blockages and obstacles that have been building up in the person's systems and energy field over time.

Such blockages and obstacles in energy can result in symptoms and dis-ease in any or all four of our bodies. For example, imagine the blockage of energy that may build up over time in our spiritual body and in our chakras if we have been experiencing the incoming of powerful spiritual energy, but have been unaware of, hiding, suppressing, or otherwise preventing this energy from flowing in a balanced, clear way. As we know, chronic or severe anxiety can be a common symptom of this type of energy gridlock, especially in those with strong psychic or mediumship gifts. Indeed, many of my clients have reported not only experiencing an alleviation of their symptoms after an energy healing, but also an emergence or intensification of their spiritual gifts.

Different healers may use different colors of light for healing. For the purpose of an energy healing, I call upon and visualize the channeling of God's gold and white light. As part of a healing, I also sometimes see colors in the recipient's body or aura, to indicate for me where they may have blockages or dis-ease in need of special attention. In addition, I may see colors around the individual to indicate strong spiritual gifts, such as purple for psychic and mediumship abilities or green for healing gifts.

Things One, Two, and Three

The thought process I use to facilitate an energy healing for an individual is a detailed one, and is often tailored to the individual who is seeking the healing, depending upon what his or her areas of need may be. For the purpose of this book, to help you learn to do an energy healing for yourself, I will be providing you with a specific meditation at the end of this chapter. But first, I would like to share with you three easy but important steps that help form the very foundation of my approach to energy healing. These three steps are taken before the healing begins.

One: I surround, ground, and shield. Before I facilitate an energy healing for an individual, I first do my own exercises to connect spiritually, protect, ground, and balance myself. This step is essential for me to do before I seek to help someone else.

Two: I call in my spirit guides and master teachers, the soul of the recipient who is seeking to be healed, and the spirit guides and master teachers of the recipient to participate in the healing. I also ask God's archangels to aid in facilitating the healing with me.

Three: I set my intention. I use my thoughts to ask God to be a channel for His gold and white light, love, and healing energy for the highest good of the recipient and all concerned. I also call upon my own sense of compassion—an extension of love, a simple desire to help—to participate in the healing process. Importantly, although I am participating in the healing, the energy I am channeling to provide the healing is not my own. It is the energy of God or the Universal Life Force. If I were using only my own energy, I would quickly become depleted. In contrast, in channeling God's love, light, and energy, both the recipient and I become the beneficiaries of the healing.

Once these initial steps are taken and my intention is set, I proceed. I place my hands over the person's head and use my thoughts to imagine a beam of God's gold and white light being sent into the top of the person's head, working through all their systems, all the way to the bottoms of their feet and into the earth—grounding, balancing, and healing them as the light flows through them. In my case, I use the power of visualization to picture this in my mind's eye. I actually see what I refer to as a jet stream of God's gold and white light and healing energy pouring into me, through me, and into and through the recipient.

Depending on the person's health issues or concerns, I may also tailor my approach to focus more intensively on a specific area of the body. A few examples are shown for you here. For all of these examples, I use my thoughts to send the intention and to picture it in my mind's eye. But again, if you cannot picture it, this is okay. Just send the intention.

- FOR ANXIETY AND PANIC ATTACKS. I imagine that the person's mind is as calm as a crystal-clear lake with no ripples.
- FOR BRAIN AND NEUROLOGICAL SYMPTOMS, INCLUDING ADD, ADHD, AND OCD. I imagine

wires with frayed segments being coated and made smooth. I picture all of the wire endings being reconnected appropriately, functioning with calm and ease.

- **FOR HEART PROBLEMS.** I may imagine a number of different things, depending on the issue. If the arteries are clogged, I picture all the gunk and plaque lining the arteries being dissolved, turned into light, and released safely out of the system, opening and making clear all blood vessels. If the issue is a flap or hole in the heart, I picture this opening getting smaller and smaller until it is closed.
- **FOR DIS-EASE OF INTERNAL ORGANS.** I imagine the ocean waves bringing their cleansing saltwater on the way into the organ and turning all toxins into light as they recede. I also imagine the shrinking of any tumors that may be present.
- **FOR INFECTION.** I imagine the affected area being filled with light and the infected cells being transformed into light and released from the body as new, healthy cells are replacing them in the body.
- **FOR BLOOD CONDITIONS.** I imagine a finely threaded net or cheese cloth being skimmed over a pool of water. The cheese cloth is filtering and purifying the blood: dissolving and transforming into light and releasing any malignant, viral, bacterial, fungal, or other abnormal cells from the bloodstream and body.

It is important to note that the intention for a healing should not be to "take away" or "get rid of" or "send away" the symptoms, dis-ease, pain, or suffering. This can actually be dangerous. We do not want dis-ease, suffering, or negativity simply to move from the recipient to the healer or to elsewhere in the Universe. Rather, the intention should be to restore balance and to heal, with the intention for the highest good of the recipient and all concerned. In this way, dis-ease, imbalance, or negativity is not transferred, but rather is *transformed* into light and love and redistributed into the earth for positive use.

The way healing manifests is different for different people. I have had many clients who have had anxiety, panic, phobias, fear, depression, migraine, pain, and other symptoms dissipate immediately. For others, the healing may take place over hours, days, or weeks. Many people have reported that a disease went into remission. Others were able to experience an emotional healing or, in some cases, a more peaceful, pain-free passing. Depending on your soul's purpose and the lessons you are meant to learn and teach in this life, the healing you experience may be spiritual, mental, emotional, physical, or some or all of the above.

In my practice, I usually do not recommend that the energy healing be done on an ongoing basis. I often tell my clients who feel well and wish to come back for maintenance purposes that this is not needed. Used in combination with their homework tools to maintain their daily health and healing (chapters 5 to 9), many people find that one energy healing is sufficient. However, if they begin to experience a re-emergence of symptoms or other difficulty, they may benefit from a tune-up healing from time to time. In addition, if someone is dealing with a longtime chronic or an advanced dis-ease, I will provide more than one healing session if needed.

Getting You Started

Through God, the power to heal resides in you. This means that you can do an energy healing for yourself. I believe in utilizing this power with integrity and care, in a responsible, protected, and balanced fashion. To get you started in learning how to do an energy healing for yourself, I am not going to immerse you in the elaborate, complex process that I utilize. Rather, I would like to suggest that you use the same three steps I do before I begin an energy healing for my clients—followed by a guided meditation, to help you begin to learn and implement the energy healing process. Before you start, please sit or lie down somewhere quiet and comfortable.

Here we go.

One: Do your surround-ground-shield exercises to protect and ground yourself (chapter 5). This is recommended, not only every day, but before an energy healing and before any spiritual work that you do.

Two: Ask your spirit guides, your master teachers, and your angels to join you and participate in your healing. You can also invite God's archangels to participate in your healing, as I do when I facilitate a healing.

Three: Ask God to send His white or golden light, love, and healing energy as part of this healing for your highest good and the highest good of all concerned. When you have done this, you are ready to begin the energy healing meditation.

Healing Your Body, Mind, and Spirit Meditation*

⇁ This meditation is designed to help you relax, heal, and balance your body, mind, and spirit. Sit back, close your eyes, and begin to breathe in through your nose to the count of four... hold it...and blow it out your mouth for four. Repeat, all the way in...hold it...and release the breath through your mouth completely.

→ I'd like you to imagine now a beautiful beam of golden light and healing energy coming in through the very top of your head, beginning to move slowly through your body from above to below. This light will help to remove any emotional, mental, or physical pain from your body.

→ Feel it entering your brain and filling it with this golden liquid light. Calming your mind like a crystal-clear lake with no ripples. All of your negative thoughts being healed and released.

→ Imagine the light now filling your face…your sinuses…your eyes…your ears…your skin and smoothly coating and clearing your throat like warm golden honey. Feel it now running through your neck and shoulders, releasing any pain or tension in these areas. Continuing slowly down through your arms…your wrists… your hands…and your fingers…healing and rejuvenating you as the golden light flows. Feeling so very relaxed, so calm, so peaceful.

→ Allow this warm golden liquid light to flow into your chest and your lungs, filling your heart and healing your heart. Letting go of all of the emotional pain and hurts, releasing them now…There is so much peace in your body now as the golden light continues to heal all of the large muscles in your upper back as well as your lower back. Feeling the light as it heals and corrects any misalignments in your spinal column and discs…

→ Filling your abdomen now as it continues to heal your body, cleansing and clearing all of your organs, relaxing you more and more.

- → Flowing gently now into your hips and all the way down your body, filling your legs...your feet...and finally, your toes.
- → All of the soreness and tensions from your body have been released into the Universe for positive distribution, as well as any toxins that have been stored in your body. Feeling your body now as it regenerates and rejuvenates. Allowing for total peace and serenity....
- → And simply now...by closing your hands into a fist and slowly, gently opening your eyes, come back into the space where you began, knowing you are better for having done this.

While the energy healings I facilitate are often done one time or on an infrequent basis, it's okay to do this meditation for yourself as often as you feel you need it. In addition, if you would like, you can add to it some of the tailored specifications for certain healing issues—like the imaginings I shared on picturing your mind as a calm, clear lake with no ripples to ease anxiety. You can also develop your own similar imaginings tailored to your situation, as long as they are done with the intention for healing and the highest good. But it's also okay if you don't want to do all of this additional "imagining." You can simply send your intention, asking to be a channel of God's love, light, and healing for your highest good. Because it's always about love.

---

*This meditation can be done as often as needed. You can also find this guided meditation on "Guided Meditations with Pat Longo" on iTunes, Amazon, and other digital platforms.

Indeed, once you are able to take all of the steps we have discussed to help you heal and maintain a healthy, balanced state of being, this healing in turn will support your opening to and loving more of yourself, including your spiritual gifts, and will lead to even more healing.

So then . . . are you ready to open your intuitive gifts and meet the whole you?

~

CHAPTER 9

Discovering and Learning to Understand Your Gift of Intuition

W E ALL HAVE IN OUR hearts our own God-given hopes, dreams, and gifts to open to, to aid us in fulfilling our soul's purpose on earth. For each of us, our paths will be different, and our gifts, including our spiritual gifts, uniquely our own. I believe these spiritual gifts—including those of a psychic, psychic mediumship, and spiritual healing nature— are facilitated by our underlying gift of intuition. Using our superpowers of intention, imagination, and intuition, we can move mountains—and anxiety.

So many of my clients and students discovered their intuition and related spiritual gifts only after spending years with anxiety, panic attacks, phobias, feelings of sadness or depression, headaches, and other symptoms. Many would tell me that they didn't want to live anymore. Most were empaths who didn't know how to protect and ground themselves spiritually. Many had no idea they were suppressing especially strong or heightened gifts of intuition. Others knew they had these abilities, but did not know how to set the spiritual boundaries to take care of themselves. Over time, it became clear to me that part of *my* soul's purpose is not only to help those who suffer with illness, but also to teach others how to love and heal themselves—and this means discovering, expressing, and realizing fully their own gift of intuition, their own truth and purpose. This, I believe, is the ultimate healing.

As we know, I believe intuition is our innate ability to sense, know, feel, or otherwise perceive not through our human experience or the normal range of our five physical senses—but through our connection to our own spiritual selves and to God and the Universe around us. Some would call this an extrasensory perception.

When we meet someone and feel as though we have known and loved them forever, this is an intuitive sense of feeling or knowing. We didn't review their résumé. We didn't interview their friends and family. We just know. When we encounter an individual and have that foreboding brick-wall or push-back feeling in our gut, or an inner voice that says caution, or the hair on the back of our neck stands up, this is also an intuitive sense of feeling or knowing. We are tuning in to the energy around that person. We all have this intuitive ability to connect and communicate with God, our spiritual selves, and the energy around us—including the spirit world.

In my experience, very few people have any idea they have spiritual gifts. But we all have a spiritual self and we all possess the gift of intuition. It's just a matter of to what degree this gift is developed and how it will manifest in us. I often refer to the expression of our intuition and related spiritual gifts as being similar to playing the piano. We can all learn to play and enjoy the piano. Some of us, like Mozart, pull up the piano bench and, with little or no effort, are off and composing symphonies. Some of us will practice, practice, practice, and our ability will reveal itself and grow in strength over time. The same is true for our intuition and the spiritual gifts through which it manifests. Each of us may have stronger natural abilities in some areas than in others.

For all of us, working to become aware of, care for, and develop our intuition and related spiritual gifts is important and will help us to live our best and most fulfilled lives. Learning to tune in to our intuition will help us to listen to our own inner voice or feeling, continue to heal ourselves, and help support the areas where we feel called to serve—perhaps in being the best parent, friend, artist, teacher, health professional, or whatever path we choose in this life.

For those of us who are suffering with spiritually based anxiety, panic, feelings of sadness or depression, frequent headaches, and other symptoms, our gift of intuition is likely quite strong—and protecting and developing this gift can be tremendously beneficial for our health and well-being. This is because our anxiety is being caused, at least in part, by external energy that is coming into our own energy field, without being recognized, controlled, or used or released in a balanced way. Without setting spiritual boundaries, the energy often will keep coming and coming unless and until the "communication" is understood or acknowledged in some way. And with nowhere to go, this persistent, unchanneled energy ultimately surfaces as anxiety and other symptoms. But when we become aware, we can set boundaries, learn to recognize this incoming energy, and develop positive channels to express, release, and use it for the purpose of good.

In my experience, those who suffer with this type of anxiety and related symptoms tend to be those whose intuitive ability is especially strong in perceiving and receiving energy that is coming to them or being communicated to them from the surrounding Universe—including beings and energies from the spirit world. This is a type of intuitive ability that would be related to having especially strong spiritual gifts of psychic or psychic mediumship abilities.

People whose gifts are especially strong in the area of spiritual healing also use their intuitive abilities. However, I have found that this type of spiritually based chronic anxiety is less common in those whose gifts manifest primarily as spiritual healing. I am not sure why this is, but I have noticed that those with strong healing abilities tend to have more grounded, balanced energy. (So stay tuned for the answer on that one.) With that said, many people have strong psychic, mediumship, *and* spiritual healing abilities—and spiritually based anxiety and other symptoms are also common in these individuals.

In this chapter, we will focus on discovering and developing our intuitive abilities, with the intention of opening to our whole selves, further alleviating anxiety and other symptoms being caused by a lack of awareness or a suppression of these intuitive gifts, and continuing our healing process. The foundation of this work will be our thoughts, using our other two superpowers of intention and imagination, with modalities such as meditation, visualization, and others to strengthen our connection to and communication with our spiritual selves and the spirit world in a way that is balanced, safe, and responsible.

How Does All This Intuition Stuff Work?

This is an excellent question—and a big one! Just how is someone able to know things that are seemingly impossible to know? How is one able to communicate with someone's loved one who has passed? Is it like a telephone call? How do we know it's real? And how is a spiritual healer able to channel God's light and love to bring healing to a recipient? I am not sure anyone has the answers to all of these questions, but I can tell you that, in my experience, it's about our nature as Divine, spiritual beings...and about energy.

Because we are all energy, we are all connected! While you and I may appear as separate individuals, in fact our energy is constantly moving and intermingling. We originated as spiritual beings and continue to be spiritual beings in physical form. I often think of us as individual cups of water, all having come from and remaining a part of the same vast ocean. We are individual souls, but from and of the same God or source. Thoughts and feelings also are energy, and like water in the ocean or like the air we breathe, constantly moving. This applies to human beings, animals, plants, and other energies on earth.

But this concept does not end with those of us in the physical world. Many of us have heard the law of physics (first law of thermodynamics) that states: "Energy cannot be created or destroyed, it can only be transferred or converted from one form to another." I am not a physicist, but I agree! I believe that when we pass from this earth, we simply shed our physical bodies and continue to live on in spirit form. Those in spirit form exchange their presence, thoughts, and feelings with us, as we do with them. I also believe that those in spirit generally carry a much higher vibration of energy than we do in physical form. My friend medium Kim Russo once used a different type of water metaphor to explain this to me—noting that H_2O can exist in different forms including ice, liquid, or vapor just as we can exist in physical or spirit form. All are the same element, the same energy, but in different forms, operating at different vibrations.

This is important because when people communicate with those on the other side, they are able to do so because they are perceiving or receiving those presences, thoughts, and feelings from the spirit world. They are intermingling with the energy of those in spirit form or the thoughts and impressions they have sent. I have found that very gifted psychics and psychic mediums are able to match and hold the vibration of their energy to that of the spirit so that they can communicate with each other effectively. Every one of us can do this to some degree. Those who are especially gifted in this area, if they accept their abilities, can do so more consistently, consciously, clearly, and for longer periods of time.

We are all on a journey to learn and grow in order to evolve as souls: to raise our level of consciousness, I believe, to that of love. This is true for souls who are in spirit form as well as physical form. For beings who are in spirit form, there exist several levels of energy or spiritual evolvement. While there is a great deal we do not know about this, in general, I refer to Level 1 as the lowest level of evolvement, carrying the lowest spiritual vibration. Level 1 represents beings in spirit form who have no remorse for the past hurts they have caused or who have chosen not to learn or evolve further. Similarly, the higher numerical levels represent higher levels of spiritual evolvement and carrying higher energetic vibrations. These are souls who strive for and demonstrate wisdom, compassion, non-judgment, mercy, grace, and all the many forms of love.

As you develop your gift of intuition and, for some of you, begin to communicate more with the spirit world, the role of your spirit guides will be essential. In addition to watching over us and providing us with guidance in our day-to-day lives, our spirit guides help us in the development and sharing of our spiritual gifts. For example, for psychics and mediums who communicate with or exchange energy with beings in spirit form, their spirit guides are important in helping them to protect their energy and space, and bring in the spirits who have messages for people in a safe, orderly, and efficient manner. It is important for them to ask their spirit guides to allow the presence of and communication with only those beings who are at a Level 2 or higher of spiritual evolvement. Souls who are choosing to stick to Level 1 are not permitted.

When we use our intuitive abilities to communicate and to receive information from the Universe, including from the spirit world, we can do so using several modes of intuition, or *extrasensory perception*. Some of us may have strengths in one or more of these senses or may experience them to a heightened degree. For those who are gifted psychics, mediums, and healers—and indeed for everyone—these forms of perception represent ways they are communicating or transmitting information or energy. These forms of perception may include any of the following:

- **CLAIRVOYANCE** = clear vision, a clear seeing from spirit. This may be experienced as a vision outside yourself, similar to the way you see other humans. More commonly, this may be something you see in your mind's eye. Either way, it can often manifest as an image, movement in your peripheral vision, flittering lights or sparkles, bright lights, blurry vision, cloudiness, auras (energy field that surrounds all living things), orbs (spheres of light), shadows, a video or movie clip, or an actual spiritual form. Often, the sighting is brief, like a flash that appears and vanishes "before your eyes." Many people do not recognize their gift of clairvoyance because they are expecting that such a gift would involve seeing a full 3-D phantom standing in front of them. Or they dismiss images they see in their mind's eye as their own old memories. But visual messages can be more subtle— and old memories and experiences are often exactly what the spirit world will show you in order to com- municate a message. For those who are primarily spiritual healers, they may see colors, auras, or other visual messages to help them identify an area of dis- ease or imbalance in the body.

- CLAIRAUDIENCE = clear hearing or listening from spirit. This can be experienced as hearing voices, words, or low-level chatter or mumbling in your ear. It can be heard from outside, like you hear other hu- mans, or from inside (as if hearing with your mind's ear). These can be messages you hear in another's voice, but most often, a message from spirit will come in your own quiet inner voice. It can even come to you as an auditory memory from your past, or as a melody or song lyric. Clairaudience can also manifest as ring- ing, high-pitched, or tunnel or underwater sounds in your ear. These sounds can be spirit trying to tune you in. So when a random song or phrase pops into your head, it indeed may be more than your memory at work.

- CLAIRSENTIENCE = clear sensing or feeling from spirit. We all have this ability, but empaths will feel the energies of others especially acutely. This can be experienced as a natural instinct or gut feeling. It can warm us with love. It can warn us of danger. It can cue us in to the thoughts, feelings, and intentions of oth- ers. It can alert us to the presence of a visitor from the spirit world. Clairsentience can also be experienced by people with psychic and mediumship abilities, when they sense a communication from spirit by feeling in their physical body. For example, they may feel their chest tighten or have trouble breathing when communicating with a deceased loved one who died by heart or lung disease. I believe clairsentience can also include the sensation of touch from spirit. Have you ever felt someone tap you on the shoulder, but when you turned around, no one was there? Touched by an angel, perhaps?

• CLAIRGUSTANCE = clear tasting from spirit. This is a taste that is experienced when you are not physically eating or drinking something. The taste can be perceived from outside, or from inside the mind. This could be as simple as a taste memory—like your grandma's pancakes—to tell you she is near. I have also known people who taste certain things as warnings. For example, one woman would taste blood in her mouth when there had been an accident or injury in the family. We also see spiritual healers who use the gift of clairgustance to help determine in what area a person may need healing. For example, they may experience a certain taste to tell them a person has liver dis-ease, another taste to let them know to look for heart dis-ease. The taste they experience corresponds with a specific part of the body or dis-ease type.

• CLAIRALIENCE OR CLAIROLFACTION = clear smelling from spirit. Like clairvoyance, clairaudience, and clairgustance, this gift is manifest by using a sensory perception, in this case the sense of smell, to bring messages or guidance. The smell can be perceived from outside, or from inside the mind (you guessed it, via the mind's nose). Indeed, we might also *smell* grandma's pancakes and know she is near. Some people smell a loved one's favorite flower or cologne. One woman I know smells flowers as an indication that someone is going to pass way: the stronger the smell, the closer the relative. In my case, I often smell my husband's cigarette smoke and know he is with me.

- **CLAIRCOGNIZANCE** = clear knowing from spirit, a sense of just knowing something. This is manifest as a knowing something or someone that you have no earthly way of knowing. It can be a sense of the past, present, or future. It can be a knowing related to the intentions of a particular person. It can be a sense of medical intuition—of knowing about an illness or area in need of healing. It can be knowledge of world events, or of universal truths. When you have the gift of claircognizance, you *just know*.

I consider these modes of extrasensory perception to be modes of intuition. They can be used to sense or communicate messages or to aid in our spiritual work. For example, as part of my work as a spiritual healer, I am blessed with claircognizance in that I have a sense of knowing information about someone's health condition, and I experience clairvoyance in that I see auras and colors around the person, which can be indicative of that individual's health, energy, and gifts. I first began to notice auras many years ago, out of the blue, when I was just beginning as a healer. I was driving along and I suddenly began to see energy fields around all of the trees on the side of the road. A clear, vibrant, white light encasing every trunk, branch, and leaf. And then one day, I caught a glimpse of my daughter's aura—a vision in beautiful bright turquoise—as she stood atop the staircase. So too, when I am teaching clients and students, I often observe the color purple around people who have a particularly heightened gift of mediumship (violet for those whose gift is developing, and deep purple for those with well developed gifts) and the color green around those having a strong gift of healing. For many people, I see both purple and green, because they possess both gifts. I also see colors related to an individual's spiritual, mental, emotional, and physical state to help guide me in my healing session. (While I have these abilities and the gift of spiritual healing, I do not practice as a medium. My abilities as a healer allow me to identify these gifts and to guide and teach people in developing their own intuitive gifts, whatever they may be. I am also grateful to have had the expertise of gifted mediums and authors, such as Kim Russo, Laura Lynne Jackson, and others, stop by on occasion to share their experiences with my class.)

All of us—including all highly gifted psychics, mediums, and healers—use one or more (usually more) of these modes of extrasensory perception or intuition to help us to connect, receive, communicate, and transmit information from the Universe around us. But what's the difference between a psychic, medium, and spiritual healer—what do they actually do?

Psychics

The term "psychic" is one that is well known but often misunderstood. We all have some degree of psychic ability. Someone who works as a psychic, sometimes also called a "spiritual psychic," "psychic intuitive," or an "intuitive," is someone who possesses a heightened sense of perception such that he or she is able to see, hear, feel, taste, smell, and/or simply know information that is provided not by the normal range of our ordinary five senses or by our sense of logic (although spirit can be quite logical), but by a connection with their spiritual selves and the energy of the Universe. He or she is able to tap into the energy around a person, animal, place, or thing and tune in to and receive information or messages that the Universe, including the spirit world, has made available or would like to communicate. These messages can apply to the present, past, or future in earth time. These messages can be related to human life, to beings in spirit form, or to the ways of the Universe. They can be practical, pertaining to day-to-day life or can be quite biblical. I often think of psychics like satellite dishes, tuning into and picking up information, "data," and communications from the Universe around us. This can include the use of any one or all of the "clair" perceptive abilities, and can include tuning in to information or beings on earth, from those in spirit, or even related to world events. Indeed, I believe the gift of having premonitions or predicting the future (sometimes referred to as prophecy), is also a psychic ability. Psychic information can come in the wake state, or during sleep (dreams, messages).

Mediums

A medium, sometimes also called a "spiritual medium" or "psychic medium," is a type of psychic. Not all psychics are mediums, but all mediums are psychics. This does not mean that a medium is more gifted than a psychic who is not a medium. It just means that mediumship is a particular type of psychic ability. Like psychics, mediums possess a heightened sense of perception such that they are able to see, hear, feel, taste, smell, and/or simply know things beyond the normal range of our five human senses. Mediums also have the heightened ability to communicate directly with beings in the spirit world, including loved ones who have passed, *in a consistent, sustained manner*. We can all communicate with beings in the spirit world to varying degrees, and psychics certainly do communicate with and receive messages from the spirit world. But mediums can do this more consistently and for longer periods of time. Often, they will not only receive information, but will have an interactive dialogue, asking questions and receiving responses. To do this, a medium must raise his or her energetic vibration to match that of the being in spirit form and maintain that connection, that shared level of energy, consistently, consciously, and for a prolonged period of time in order to convey an accurate and complete message. Professional psychics and mediums may choose to deliver their messages as part of a special session for the recipient, often referred to as a "reading."

Spiritual Healers

We all have the power to heal within us. I believe we all also have the ability to formulate a healing intention for the highest good, and send love, light, and healing light to others. But some of us have a particularly strong ability in this area. I believe healers are people who were born to earth to respond to and alleviate suffering. Often, we see healers in the helping professions like physicians, nurses, social workers, therapists, hospice workers, teachers, and clergy. These are people whose souls want to reach out and eliminate the pain—to balance and restore in spirit, mind, heart, and body. Often, their healing work takes place through these traditional jobs or venues. Some of us are called to the path of spiritual healing. Spiritual healing is sometimes also referred to as "energy healing," "natural energy healing," "faith healing," "hands-on healing," and other terms.

Spiritual healing consists of the provision of care to the spiritual body, working to facilitate the healing of the spirit in order to restore balance and, for many, to achieve healing also in the mental, emotional, and physical bodies. Spiritual healers can use any number of techniques, including energy healing, reiki, therapeutic touch, and many others. They can use intuition, or extrasensory perception—such as seeing, hearing, feeling, tasting, smelling, and knowing—to guide and help facilitate their healing work. I believe that spiritual healers are here to work in collaboration with (not instead of) our health professionals—like physicians, nurses, and therapists— to provide care to the whole person for the highest good.

Even among those psychics, mediums, and healers who are blessed with exceptionally strong or heightened abilities, no gift is the same. We are all unique, with our own individual blueprint. Different people experience different forms of perception. Some see spirits, while others may see a scene in their heads as though watching a video. Many hear messages in their own voices, inside their own mind's ear. Some experience or feel a physical sensation of how a loved one passed or feel a loved one's love for us. Some may actually feel transported to another place and time, while they watch or feel an incident occur and then relay it to the client.

In addition, different people may use different techniques to "tune in" or facilitate the communication process. For example, some psychics and mediums may use scribbling or tarot cards to help focus their ability to receive and then give a message. Some may use automatic writing, putting pen to paper, asking the spirit world a question, and observing what comes out in the writing. Often this writing is done with great speed and in someone else's handwriting. Some may use psychometry, or holding an object, photo, or a client's hand to pick up energy while they "read." Still others may get up and walk the room, which helps them to move the energy, while receiving and giving their messages.

So too, the ways in which a spiritual healer works are as varied as the number of healers themselves. Some have a sense of knowing about a client's health, some see beings in spirit form, some hear words or voices, some literally experience a sense of smell or taste to diagnose illness. Some use touch, others don't. In my case, I work as an energy healer with a faith in God. I do the surround-ground-shield and additional extensive grounding exercises, and then ask to be a channel of God's healing light, love, and energy for the highest good of the recipient and all concerned. I use other abilities, like clairvoyance and claircognizance, to help guide the healing effort. I often feel my hands heat up when someone in need of healing has been placed in my path. As the healing process occurs, my entire body will often heat up significantly. Some healers will experience this type of "heating up," visions, or other sensations as they perform a healing, while others may not sense anything like this at all.

Many people have a combination of these spiritual gifts and abilities, and each has taken a different path to discover them. I have found many, many people who had strong intuitive gifts that they had not yet discovered—and it has usually been those who possess a strong sense of intuition of the psychic or psychic mediumship type who suffer with spiritually based anxiety and related symptoms. Perhaps you or your loved one could be one of them.

Could This Be You?

How do we know whether having extreme intuitive abilities is a part of us, or even as part of the reason we suffer with anxiety and other symptoms? As we will see from the stories Carol, Dorene, Steven, MaryAnn, Diana, and Eileen have graciously agreed to share here, the finding out is often as unique as the gifts themselves. While we are all different, you just might see yourself in them.

Carol (Ofenloch) Tranchina

Let's start by saying I have known my younger sister Carol all of her life. Did I know she was a spiritual medium, way back when? I had no idea.

I remember Carol as being sad through much of her childhood. She was shy and introverted. In school, she was afraid to raise her hand or speak out in class. She usually had only one close friend. I remember when Carol was in the first or second grade, my sisters and I frequently would be called out of our classes to console her, as she would inevitably be in tears for some reason or other. She seemed afraid of her own shadow, and none of us knew why. As an adult, Carol became very successful in her job but she still did not like to speak in meetings or in front of other people.

I now know that Carol is an empath, and all that time, she was experiencing other people's feelings, energy, and emotion. She also saw spirits in our family home, which terrified her. She saw and heard and felt things whenever she went out into the world. She also would inadvertently predict the future. In one case, she remembers being in the third or fourth grade, telling people all about our dog who had puppies. She told them about the number of pups in the litter and what they all looked like from nose to tail. As it turns out, the dog had not had puppies. But sure enough, some months later, that dog gave birth to the exact number of puppies Carol had foretold and they looked exactly how she had described them. On a day-to-day basis, Carol saw and heard and felt things that she did not understand. She felt like an outsider, like she didn't belong, even in her own family. She thought she was crazy, and can recall often telling herself, out loud, "Carol, stop talking to yourself."

Fast-forward a few decades later. I had become a spiritual healer and teacher—pretty much out of the blue—and was offering weekly classes in my home. The classes focused on enhancing our spiritual connection and, among other things, discovering and embracing our spiritual gifts. While Carol did not attend my class initially, she had a friend she thought might enjoy it and accompanied her one day. In the end, Carol is the one who continued coming to class. She says that, finally, she felt like she belonged. Many of the students were able to recognize that they had certain spiritual gifts, such as psychic, mediumship, or healing abilities. Carol did too. But of course, she did not say anything. When she finally started to share her messages, it was clear to me that she was a medium!

When Carol began providing readings for people, she was able to see how helpful and healing the messages were to those who received them. She began working as a professional medium, giving readings not only to individuals, but also to groups, to dozens of people at a time. As she began to realize and accept this as a part of herself, her symptoms subsided. Her anxiety and sadness went away. Her fear of speaking disappeared. At long last, Carol felt like herself.

Dorene Bair

Dorene is our extra Longo child, our honorary member of the family. She has been the best friend of my daughter Christine since they were thirteen years old. I had no idea at the time, but as a child, Dorene often had thoughts and feelings that scared and confused her. She frequently felt that people were angry or upset with her. She felt outside of things. She says she had always felt a spiritual connection, but was not aware of having spiritual gifts. It was not until she was twenty-six, after the breakup with a longtime boyfriend, that her spiritual journey began to open up before her.

I remember Dorene, my daughter Christine, and I were on an airplane on our way to a kickline event in Florida. Dorene was feeling very low, as the relationship with her boyfriend of nine years, the man she had hoped to marry, had ended. So I reached up to her in the seat in front of me and handed her a little book of spiritual affirmations. She liked the book, and so I invited her to join me at my teacher Holly's next spiritual awareness class.

Dorene soon discovered that she is an empath and has the gift of mediumship through automatic writing, channeling, and remote viewing. Indeed, the first time Dorene joined Holly's class, we were given an exercise to tune in intuitively to another person in the room. Dorene immediately connected with the energy of a woman in class and began to pick up that this woman was concerned about a certain young man. Dorene quickly connected with this gentleman's energy and was able to "remote view" a moment in time with him.

This means she was able to view and experience that moment, as though she were experiencing it herself. She could see the cornfields outside of his window, she could sense that he just wanted to be left alone, and that he was heavily medicated. The woman validated all of these details.

A short time later, Dorene, my nephew Steven, my daughter Tricia, my friend Kim Russo,, and I started our own little spiritual awareness class. Around this time (and pretty much from then on), Dorene's gift of automatic writing took off like a rocket ship. We began keeping a journal and writing down thoughts as they came to us. For Dorene, this exercise was like a natural reflex. She would hear "pick up the pen" and off she would go. Amazingly, the writings Dorene would receive would appear in handwriting that was not her own. In fact, her first automatic writing came from a friend's sister who was in the spirit world. Her friend confirmed all the details that were provided in the message, and also noted that the handwriting was her sister's! From there, Dorene proceeded to channel writings from her spirit guides and from many people's loved ones who had passed. Many of her writings were from a spirit guide who called himself Stephanos, who provided universal messages with love and healing for all. His signature, which he included at the end of each message, would always appear exactly the same.

And so at the age of twenty-six, Dorene had discovered that she was an empath—that all of those sad, scary, and confusing feelings she had felt as a child were not her own. They were not her truth, but the truth of the persons whose energy she had been taking on. She discovered her spiritual self and began to feel normal for the first time in her life. Today, Dorene looks at life through the eyes of gratitude, thankful even for the difficult experiences that have challenged and taught her valuable lessons. She uses her intuitive gifts to teach, coach, and serve as a change agent to help others to live their highest and best lives.

Steven Hughes

Steven is my much beloved nephew. He is also a spiritual medium, healer, and teacher. As a child, Steven used to see auras around all living things. When he would draw pictures, he would incorporate these energy fields into the scene. Like so many other children, he was told by adults to stop drawing these strange things—to draw only what was real. And so, he learned to put that part of himself away. Steven also started healing others when he was about eight years old. He says that he just instinctively knew where to place his hands to help people. When he was a teenager, he would sleep with the television on deep into the night to help distract him from the whispers and shadows he would hear and see. I had no idea he was experiencing this as a young person. I would not find out until years later, after I began to follow my spiritual path and discover my own gift of healing.

Steven went on to serve in the Marines, and as a presidential guard, embassy guard, and part of a recon unit. He trained at Quantico, and became an expert in security, safety, weapons, and tactics. He wrote security plans for embassies, worked with kids who had been in jail, and later became a police officer and wrote security plans for our schools. It was while in the Marines that Steven discovered his ability as an automatic writer, which is a way of receiving and expressing messages from the spirit world. He was in the California desert training at the time, and he began hearing just one repetitious word or phrase in his head again and again. For example, he would hear "A flower needs soil and water to grow" over and over again. At first he ignored it, thinking it was just his own mind. Finally, he began to write the words down, sometimes just one single word. But as soon as he wrote this one word or phrase, more would come. What Steven didn't yet know was that he was a spiritual or psychic medium, receiving messages through automatic writing.

These experiences flashed Steven back to his childhood, to all he had heard and seen back then, and he felt validated. He called his mother, who told him, "You know, your aunt Pat is taking spiritual classes now. You should call her." He did call me, and I immediately knew he was extremely gifted and advised him in the importance of spiritual protection and balance. When Steven returned to Long Island, he began coming to some of Holly's classes, and shortly thereafter he joined Dorene, Tricia, Kim, and myself in forming our little group.

Steven's gifts as a medium and healer developed rapidly, and he was soon offering these services to others—that is, when he was not at his full-time job. Today, he practices as a spiritual healer and teacher. Steven continues to receive the most beautiful writings from God, angels, and other spiritual beings. I just cannot get enough of them and I hope, one day soon, Steven, too, will write a book!

MaryAnn DiMarco

MaryAnn and I met when she called, looking for an appointment with a spiritual medium in the hope of connecting with her loved ones who had recently passed. I immediately explained that I am not a medium, I am a spiritual healer, but as part of the healing process, I help people open up to their whole selves and learn to develop their own spiritual gifts. "I'm coming in," was MaryAnn's response. She seemed to know instantly that this was for her.

MaryAnn had known since age five or so that she had spiritual gifts. She would see things, hear things, and have dreams in which she visited with loved ones or even predicted the future. She would also experience little signs in her daily life—like singing a song in her mind and having it play on the radio seconds later, thinking of a friend she hadn't heard from in a while and receiving a call from him, or sensing danger on the road while driving. At one point she had this sense, said out loud to herself, "There's going to be a car accident," pulled over to the side of the road, and a car accident happened right in front of her. MaryAnn also reports having intuitive dreams as a child and still today as an adult. In one dream, she saw her grandmother who had passed—looking young, healthy, and dressed in an elegant black dress—only to find that her mother had had the exact same dream the exact same night. Much more recently, she had a dream in which she visited with her late father-in-law with whom she had been very close. She was at a party and she saw him there, sitting at a table. He looked wonderful. His eyes were blue and shining, his hair was cut just right, and he was wearing one of his trademark bright blue checkered shirts. He looked at MaryAnn and asked, "Please tell Elaine [his wife] about the eyes. Everything will be okay." When MaryAnn relayed this message, Elaine replied that their son was scheduled to have eye surgery—and she was comforted by her husband's words.

As MaryAnn was growing up, her mother had been a spiritualist and had been open about these abilities, the use of meditation, and the pursuit of higher consciousness. MaryAnn's mother was also highly supportive of her gifts. Perhaps because of this awareness and support from her mother, MaryAnn had not suffered with chronic anxiety or related symptoms throughout her life, like so many of my other clients and students had. But when she reached her early twenties, MaryAnn found herself searching for more information on what all of these experiences meant and how to develop and use her abilities.

In her healing session, we talked about the things in MaryAnn's life that might be causing her pain or difficulty. She had recently been through a divorce, her beloved father-in-law had died, and she was feeling grief-stricken and depressed. She was also confused about what to do with these strange intuitive experiences she had been having all of her life. When I did the energy healing for MaryAnn, she told me afterward that she had seen her father-in-law appear directly before her during the healing. He had said to her, "This is your time . . . I will be back." I was thrilled. I told MaryAnn, "You are a psychic medium!" She explained that, while she had always been able to see, hear, and feel beings in spirit form, she just didn't know how to understand or translate it into words or meaningful messages. That's when I advised her that spirit usually doesn't speak to us in a loud, booming, disembodied voice from the heavens, like in the movies. We usually hear messages from the spirit world delivered in our own, inner voice. And right then, in that moment, it all clicked for MaryAnn. I have no recollection of this, but according to MaryAnn, I then asked her if she was ready for the ride of her life! I invited her to join my spiritual awareness classes, and MaryAnn the Medium—author of *Believe, Ask, Act: Divine Steps to Raise Your Intuition, Create Change, and Discover Happiness*—has been using her gift as a psychic medium to help and heal others ever since.

Diana Cinquemani

When I met Diana, she was dedicated to being a teacher and she was very good at it. It's all she ever wanted to do and to be, but she suffered with terrible anxiety and irrational phobias, like her fear of elevators, popping balloons, and the dark. Diana was only about twenty-three years old then, when a fellow teacher told her that I might be able to help her with her anxiety. She thought, even though she had no idea about spirit, it was worth a try. When she began my class, Diana was not expecting the journey it would take her on.

When Diana attended my class, she saw that many people with anxiety found opening to their spiritual gifts to be extremely helpful. She thought that the meditation portion of my class would be the key to bringing her peace. Though she was unsure about

where she fit in, she continued to attend class diligently for about two years.

Even though Diana loved the classes, at that point,
her life became extremely busy and she stopped coming.
About three years later, I received a phone call from
Diana, after her aunt had approached her about resum-
ing her "angel classes." Though her meditation practice
was very beneficial, Diana told me she had just had a
rough three years and knew something was missing.
When she began to attend my classes regularly again, it
became apparent to me that she was a psychic medium.
However, Diana was determined to continue teaching—
after all, it's all she had ever wanted. She just didn't see
herself being a professional psychic or medium. I truly
believe in allowing my students to let their gift unfold
in Divine timing, and so I wanted Diana to come into
her gift when she was ready.

Then one day, she made an appointment with me
for a healing session, to try to work more on her anxiety and fear issues. I did a past-life regression for her,
because in many people, hurts and irrational fears also
can come from experiences from past lives. In the regression, she was able to identify and release the
sources of her fear of elevators and popping sounds. At
the end of the regression, she had a unique experience
of seeing and feeling her third-eye chakra expanding
and filling with the color purple. She came out of the
regression, feeling a magnificent peace. She truly
thought that was the end of her journey with me and
she accomplished what she had come to class for. However, the very next day, her mediumship abilities could
no longer be suppressed. They exploded. Diana called
me in a panic, seeing and hearing way too much. She

came in to see me immediately, and we began working on helping her to protect herself and set boundaries more effectively. From there, she began using the needed tools to help her to connect, ground, and protect herself spiritually.

As with many gifted individuals, Diana is an empath as well as a psychic medium. This means in addition to deriving anxiety from her past-life fears, her symptoms were also coming from both picking up and absorbing the energies around her as an empath and from suppressing the spiritual energy that she was receiving and perceiving as a psychic medium. When she began using the surround-ground-shield exercises, she was able to reduce the intake and absorption of the energies around her and alleviate the anxiety associated with this. To eliminate her anxiety completely, I advised her she would also need to accept and share her gift of mediumship. Unsure, Diana slowly began to use her gifts only in class, but wasn't ready to share them with the world.

When Diana turned thirty, she was excessed from her current teaching position, even though the kids and everyone at the school loved her. She found herself in a waiting period from September to January until another position became available. I told her that there was something else she was meant to be doing. I asked her to come and provide readings to the others in my class and she did—making one lady cry, happy tears of course, as she relayed a message from a loved one in the spirit world. Diana approached me after class with a question: "How do I know where this is all coming from? How do I know that I'm not making all of this up?"

"Why would you make it up?" I asked, knowing that, in Diana's case, she was not.

"I would never," she said emphatically.

Exactly my point.

And that was that. Shortly thereafter, Diana came to me and told me that there might be something to this. She thought she was, after all, a psychic medium. I told her, with a heavy dose of sarcasm, that I was relieved it had only taken seven years for her to realize this. Very quickly, Diana chose not to return to teaching and began working as a full-time professional psychic medium. She is a highly gifted reader, providing messages from spirit guides and loved ones, as well as a kind of "soul mapping," helping people to identify and live their soul's purpose. She has accepted her whole self and is sharing her gift just as she was meant to do, with very little anxiety.

Eileen Kelly

From the time she was a little girl, Eileen just knew things. People would come to her with their problems and concerns and, often, she would advise them. She was wise beyond her years—and also extremely gifted. While Eileen knew she had *something* going on, it would be decades before she would realize the extent of her gift.

In many ways, Eileen's childhood was ideal, with two wonderful parents who loved each other and their four children. However, she struggled with her weight and with severe asthma. At that time, the treatment options for asthma were more limited and her father would frequently need to rush her to the emergency room, where doctors would give an adrenaline injection and nebulizer therapy to open her airways. It seemed they were going to the hospital every day. There were many close calls, but there was one that had a particularly significant impact on her life.

Eileen was eight years old. She and her father were in the car, with Eileen in respiratory distress and her father driving as fast as he could to get her to the hospital. He would periodically pull the car over to give her mouth-to-mouth resuscitation. Even though this is not especially helpful for an asthma attack, he didn't know what else he could do. When they arrived at the emergency room, the medical team took Eileen back for treatment. She still could not breathe. The last thing she remembers before everything went black is screaming, "I'm going to die. I'm going to die. I'm going to die." The next thing she recalls is waking up in her hospital bed. Everyone told her that she had nearly died. She wondered whether indeed she had died and come back to life. She didn't know, but shortly after this incident, she seemed to develop an enhanced sense of intuition. She would see and hear things that others didn't—and she just sort of knew things that she had no earthly way of knowing.

As Eileen entered into her teen and young adult years, her dream was to have what her parents had. She wanted to be married and have a family, and she had thought she had met the man with whom she would spend her life. At twenty-four, when that relationship ended, she was devastated. Even though it was for the best, at the time it seemed like the end of the world. A few months later, with Eileen still recovering from her recent breakup, her father became ill and passed away suddenly. It was a devastating loss. Eileen and her siblings were heartbroken. Her mother was inconsolable. Eileen continued to work in her job and, after a time, began dating again. But some years later, Eileen's mother also became ill and Eileen helped to take care of her during this time. Sadly, five years after her diagnosis, her mother passed away.

Still grief-stricken and feeling depressed by the loss of both parents, Eileen did her best to get back into the swing of things. She began seeing a new boyfriend. She found it nice to be dating again, but after a few months, found that she had started to close down. She no longer heard that still small voice inside. Her gift had gone silent. She had lost herself. And she began to develop terrible anxiety. While she used to enjoy going to the gym five times a week, she could no longer manage this. She would drive to the gym after work and, as soon as she stepped through the gym door, would be hit by a feeling of overwhelming anxiety and intense nausea. Every day she kept trying, but the nausea only got worse. All she could do was turn around and head back to the parking lot.

After about eleven months, Eileen decided to "take herself back" and end the relationship, which she and her boyfriend agreed wasn't the right match for either of them. As it would happen, around this same time, the daughter of Eileen's friend was planning to host a group reading with a psychic medium—and this friend kept telling Eileen that she should go. She was excited for the opportunity and decided to attend. Little did Eileen know that her friend's daughter is my niece, and the group reading was in my brother's house.

When I met Eileen, I knew immediately that she was an empath. I gave her the surround, ground, and shield exercises to help with her anxiety and nausea. I also invited her to join one of my classes. And let me tell you, Eileen is a serious student. She is hilariously funny, but she also means business. On day one, she told me she had begun practicing surround-ground-shield immediately after our first meeting. The very day she started using these exercises, her anxiety had been eliminated. She had begun going to the gym again without issue. In class, she listened. She took notes. She did her homework. And Eileen's gift began to develop rapidly. Today, Eileen is a professional psychic medium who provides readings with the intention of bringing messages of comfort and healing. In reclaiming her gift, she says she feels whole again. Now, she is working to bring that same sense of wholeness, happiness, and love to others.

Seeing the Signs

We know that every one of us has intuitive abilities to discover and use in our lives. From these few stories, we can see how each person, each story, each gift is different and beautiful in its own way. For some, the recognition and acceptance comes quickly. For others, it takes time. For many people, the gift of intuition is largely unrealized or suppressed and that act of suppression, whether conscious or unconscious, can result in anxiety, panic, feelings of sadness, and other related symptoms. From my perspective, I just want this suffering to end. I want the symptoms to stop. I want people to feel whole. I want them to be free.

Carol, Dorene, Diana, and so many others had no idea that they were empaths or that they had these exceptional psychic intuitive abilities. They didn't know this is why they were suffering. Yet so many signs were there. Could you, like Carol and Diana, be missing the signs that you have hidden intuitive abilities in need of discovery and development? Over my years of experience, I have been able to observe lots of clues that may indicate the presence of strong intuitive gifts, lying just beneath the surface. Let's see if any of them sound like you.

Signs That Spirit May Be Communicating with You

- Do you have any of the traits of an empath (chapter 1)?
- Do you have unexplained anxiety, panic, phobias, or feelings of sadness or depression that do not respond sufficiently to medical treatment?
- Do you suffer from frequent, unexplained headaches?
- Do you sometimes feel pressure on your forehead, or third-eye chakra, or pressure like a band around your head?
- Do you have unexplained sensations in your ears—like a ringing sound, tunnel sound, or feeling of pressure?
- Inside your head, do you sometimes hear unintelligible low-level chatter in your ear?
- In your mind's eye, also called the third eye, do you sometimes see flashes of faces, videos, or other images that pop up randomly?
- Do you sometimes see things that "aren't there" in your peripheral vision?
- Do you sometimes hear songs or words in your head that pop up randomly?

- Do you ever have the sensation of smelling or tasting something from out of nowhere?
- Do you ever just know things, or have a sense of knowing, and you don't know why or how?
- Do you at times have a sense of someone or something—and then you see or hear from that someone, or that something occurs in the future?
- Do you ever feel chills running up and down your body for no reason?
- Do you sometimes feel unexplained tingling on the top of your head or down your spine?
- Do you ever have vivid dreams in which you visit with a loved one, or witness or receive information in some way?
- Do you ever know what's going to happen before it happens? Does the information you receive in your dreams or while awake ever come true in the future?

Many of these signs may seem strange—but in my world, they are quite common. I do recommend that people who have these signs or symptoms, or any others, see a doctor to rule out any physical or mental dis-ease or imbalance. It is important to care for our whole self. When looking at the spiritual self, I can tell you that these signs are common in people who have strong psychic or mediumship gifts. For example, headaches or pressure in the head can occur as spiritual energy comes into the crown and third-eye chakras. Ringing, low-level chattering, or other sounds in the ears can occur when spirit is trying to talk to us, to tune us in. We may see things that quickly appear and disappear—often in our mind's eye and often in our peripheral vision. This can be spirit trying to show themselves or show us a memory or message. The same is true with smells and tastes. The sensation of chills or goose bumps is often experienced when spirit is near, or to indicate that what was just said is true or profound. A tingling sensation from the top of the head on down can indicate the opening of the crown chakra. In addition to these experiences, I have found that people can experience a cough—almost like a strong tickle in their throat—as spirit tries to communicate a message. And of course, we have talked about the anxiety, panic attacks, and related symptoms that can emerge from the suppression or lack of awareness around these powerful gifts. Such anxiety, heart palpitations, and/or a sense of urgency can also occur as spirit is trying to give a message, and will dissipate as soon as the message is acknowledged or shared.

I wonder, do you recognize any of these signs from your own life? Do you see yourself in Carol, Dorene, Steven, MaryAnn, Diana, Eileen, or the others who have shared their stories in the pages of this book? If you do, if this is who *you* are, then this may be your story too.

CHAPTER 10

Awakening and Developing
Your Gift of Intuition

ISCOVERING OUR GIFT OF INTUITION can be exciting—
and healing. Whatever our unique gifts turn out to be,
however they manifest for us, we must commit to develop and
use them with integrity and with the intention to offer them
in love and service, for the highest good. To do this, we must
also ensure that we take care of ourselves by protecting ourselves, setting healthy boundaries, and maintaining balance in
our spiritual, mental, emotional, and physical bodies. Here,
you will begin to awaken the power within and develop your
own gift of intuition—by utilizing effective tools and techniques to strengthen your connection to spirit, enhance your
awareness of your sensory perceptions, build those intuitive
muscles, and set the ground rules to do this with balance and
integrity. In doing this, you may begin to see spiritually based
symptoms—like anxiety, panic, feelings of sadness or depression, headache, and others—begin to dissipate with the flow

of this spiritual energy and the emergence of the full truth and purpose of your soul.

First Things First: Integrity and Intention

It is important today and every day onward to commit to learning to develop and use your abilities with integrity and in a balanced, responsible manner. As part of that commitment, a few important principles are key:

- Setting your intention for the highest good
- Having faith, not fear
- Honoring yourself
- Protecting and grounding yourself
- Letting go of EGO (Edging-God-Out)

SETTING YOUR INTENTION. Before we start any activity, it is important to set our intention. Our specific intention may vary slightly, depending on the activity we are undertaking. However, our overall intention should always be to use our intuitive abilities with integrity, for the purpose of love, light, and healing in service to the highest good. Unfortunately, there are people who use their gifts for negative purposes. We want to be sure we are working with God, for *goodness'* sake.

HAVING FAITH, NOT FEAR. For those who want to develop their spiritual gifts, faith is paramount. All over the world, people are rising up into a higher spiritual consciousness. In response, we see a surge of darkness scrambling for ground anywhere it can find it. But negativity cannot exist without fear. Fear is what feeds and draws more fear, more negativity.

And in the spiritual world, this can mean beings in spirit form who have negative energy or even sinister intentions.

Before fear has a chance to occur, proactively draw on your faith and utilize the tools afforded by God's light and protection. Using the power of your thoughts, imagine the following:

- Surround yourself in God's white light and protection.
- Push God's white light out on the path ahead of you.
- Send white light into a room, or among the people with whom you will be interacting, ahead of your arrival.
- Send pink light out to people with whom you may have challenging relationships or situations.
- Send white and pink light out to the world—even to dictators, terrorists, and those who seek to cause harm in the world—for nothing but love can conquer hate. Nothing but light can conquer the dark.

If you encounter a situation in which you feel there is fear or negative energy, say the Lord's Prayer (or the preferred prayer of your faith), silently or out loud, or push God's white light throughout the entire room and beyond. Tell the energy, "Only those beings who walk in God's white light are welcome here. All negative beings, entities, or energies must leave immediately by the power of the I Am (God)."

Remember—in a space of darkness, even the smallest flame will light the entire room.

There is nothing to fear. Darkness cannot stand in the light. The light will always win.

HONORING YOURSELF. This is about loving yourself and setting boundaries to take care of yourself. For me, it was only when I said no to the overload of obligations and activities in my life, and began to say yes to the things that fed my soul, that my spiritual gifts began to emerge. When we stop to listen to and honor ourselves, we are better able to connect with our higher selves and with God. When we do this, and when we live in balance, our gifts become clearer and we are better able to love and honor others as well. This means listening to that still small voice inside, realizing what we want and what we don't want, and pursuing what we love. It does not mean abandoning our obligations to our families and others. However, neither does it mean saying yes to all invitations and all comers. We should be kind, respectful, and gracious, but we do not have to say yes to everything. Remember, place the oxygen mask on yourself before assisting others.

PROTECTING AND GROUNDING. A fundamental principle of spiritual awareness and development is to start each day with protection and grounding. This is also essential to do before any type of psychic, mediumship, or spiritual healing work. We have covered this extensively in chapters 4 and 5, but it is important to repeat here for those who are seeking to further develop their spiritual connection and abilities. Protection and grounding are essential in ensuring that we are safe and balanced, and that we are offering a safe and balanced space for others. For this reason, we should never pursue psychic, mediumship, healing, or other spiritual work or activities without first being protected, grounded, and balanced in God's white light.

SURROUND, GROUND, AND SHIELD. The practice of surround, ground, and shield is a quick process, taking all of ten seconds a day (chapter 5). In my opinion, these exercises should be done by all people, everywhere. In addition, more extensive grounding exercises are often needed for those who are doing spiritual work (try the Universal White Light Meditation for this). Because these individuals are working with spiritual energy—energy of a very high vibration—they must balance this energy by grounding to the earth. Indeed, in my experience, the more grounded we are, the higher our vibration of energy can be and the higher the vibration of energy we can work with while here on the earth.

ENERGY CLEARING. It is important to clear any negative energy from ourselves, our things, and our space regularly (see chapter 5). For most people, a space clearing of the home done every three months is sufficient. I would also recommend this exercise if you've had a guest who has come from a place where negative energies are more likely to hang out— like a bar or other environment with drinking, drugs, or spiritually high-risk activity. In addition to clearing our space, we also need to clear ourselves and any new objects (especially antiques or secondhand items) of negative energy. Because everything is made of energy, furniture, jewelry, mirrors, gems, and anything that comes from the earth stores energy. Our own persons also can be followed by spiritual "hitchhikers" if we do not protect ourselves. All of this energy can be removed through a simple clearing exercise, using the power of intention, on our persons, objects, and space whenever needed (chapter 5). For those doing spiritual work, I would recommend clearing your own person and the space where the spiritual work is being done at the end of each day.

LETTING GO OF EGO (EDGING-GOD-OUT). The "ego" may mean different things to different people. For the purpose of spiritual work, I use this term to refer to an *imbalanced* ego—

or anything coming from our own individual personality self that is not Godlike. This may include judging other people and their circumstances, holding grudges, withholding forgiveness, indulging feelings of jealousy, envy, or spite, or harboring ill intentions or motivations in our work or interactions with others. We can all experience momentary flashes of these thoughts and feelings. This is human and we need not judge ourselves for this. But instead of indulging these thoughts and feelings, we need to bring ourselves back to God and let them go.

There is no place for ego, or Edging-God-Out, in our spiritual work. When providing a message or healing to someone, it is not our job to judge them. Similarly, it's not our job to doubt the message provided by spirit or to offer our own opinion on an issue or situation. It is also not our job to try to deliver a message in a way that aggrandizes ourselves or makes us appear the most dramatic or impressive. It's our job to provide the messages from those in spirit as clearly and gently as possible, for the purpose of love and healing. To keep our ego in balance, we must connect with God, pray to have pure intention and motivation, and do the work necessary to love and heal ourselves.

Setting the Ground Rules

Before getting started in opening to and building our intuition, it's important to understand a few basics and set the ground rules for communicating with the Universe and spirit world. Living in spirituality is different from living in spirit form. As you begin to seek to connect more with those in spirit form, it's important to know that you can and should direct how and when this type of communication takes place.

GET TO KNOW YOUR SPIRIT GUIDES. We all have spirit guides assigned to us. It's important to talk with and listen to our spirit guides and to ask them for their help and guidance. You can do this in prayer or meditation. Some people will hear or see or become aware of the name of one or more of their spirit guides. Others may not feel the need to know the names and number of their guides, as long as they know they are there. Your spirit guides will help to protect you, heal you, teach you, guide you, and, when communicating with the spirit world, to set boundaries and keep order. They will give you what you can handle, a little at a time. It's important to have patience. As you learn more, you will be shown more.

SET YOUR BOUNDARIES. Those in the spirit world do not have the same sense of time and space or the same physical needs that we have. When beginning to tune in to your intuition, you will need to work with your spirit guides to set boundaries for those in spirit form—to ensure that you can eat, work, relax, spend time with your family, sleep, and be human! This is important for maintaining balance in your life and for fostering your ability to be an effective psychic, medium, or healer. If you do not honor and protect yourself, you will become depleted and your gifts, too, will lose strength and clarity. So as you work on your intuitive gifts, it's important to know that you are in charge. You have control. It is your right to communicate when you so choose to receive and give messages. You can indicate when you are and are not available for such communication by telling this to your spirit guides, so that they can put this into action for you. You can also communicate this directly to the Universe and others in spirit form. This will help you as you begin, by reducing the amount of unwanted incoming energy that you experience —and will be even more helpful as you begin to develop even greater sensitivity and stronger abilities to connect and communicate.

Here are a few important steps:

- Set your intention. Tell your spirit guides that you wish to receive only messages that will help facilitate love and healing and the highest good. Be sure to tell them you do *not* want to see death or negative events, unless you can help prevent them or bring healing to them. They will act as your protectors and orchestrate your wishes for you.

- Utilize a spiritual Do Not Disturb" sign when you are sleeping or otherwise unavailable for communication with the spirit world. Just use thought to post the sign in your mind and ask your spirit guides to help you enforce this request. You may want to include one exception to the rule—do not disturb except in the case of emergency. If there's an emergency and you and spirit can help, then you will want to know this.

- If you have designated hours when you wish to communicate with the spirit world, be specific about this. Tell your guides when you would like to communicate with the spirit world. Be sure to tell them in *earth time*, for example, Mondays, Tuesdays, and Wednesdays, 6:00 P.M.–9:00 P.M. eastern standard time, earth time.

- Use a symbol, such as the lighting of a white candle, to indicate when you are open to communicate.

- Ask your spirit guides to develop a spiritual waiting room for beings in spirit form who walk in God's white light and wish to communicate with you. You want to ask your spirit guides specifically for only those beings at an evolvement level of 2 or above—and to coordinate the messages efficiently, so that you communicate with one being at a time. Level 1 of spiritual evolvement represents beings who are negative, have not shown remorse for past hurts, or have chosen not to evolve further. Those on higher levels can communicate at a lower vibration, but those on lower levels cannot enter the higher levels until they have evolved sufficiently to do so.

- Be sure to make it clear that beings who do not walk in God's white light, negative beings, and beings from below Level 2 are *not* permitted near you or in your space. Ever.

These steps to protect and set boundaries are critical not only for adults but also for children. There are so many children who are empaths and are highly gifted spiritually. Many are suffering because they don't understand what is happening to them or know what to do about it. As adults, we need to help our children when they report that they see or hear or feel things, when they are afraid to be alone, when they develop anxiety in groups (empathic energy), or at nighttime when the visions or voices come. They need to know that this is real, but there is nothing to be afraid of. I remember speaking to one mother who was beside herself because her eleven-year-old daughter was terrified and couldn't sleep. She was seeing faces at night. They were lining up to talk to her, but she didn't understand why they were there or what they wanted. I told her mother to please tell her daughter that she does not need to be afraid, that she has control. I instructed her to tell the girl that she was to command the spirits to leave her, to say that they are not allowed in her space, that she is not ready for them yet. When I spoke to the mother sometime later, she told me they were making progress. The little girl had told the spirits to leave her room and they had all left. The only problem was, now she could not use the bathroom at night. When she opened her bedroom door, all the spirits had lined up in the hallway outside her room! This is a lesson to all of us to be clear and specific. The little girl updated her instructions, telling them to please leave *her* alone, that they are not allowed in the space where she is until further notice. She now sleeps very well and without disturbance.

For most children, it's when they enter their late teens and early adulthood that their spiritual gifts will re-emerge and begin to intensify, and they will need further guidance in learning how to set boundaries and develop their gifts in a positive, balanced way. In the meantime, parents can help their children to use the surround, ground, and shield exercises (in an age-appropriate manner) on a daily basis to protect them spiritually and manage any related anxiety. Communicating with beings in spirit form can and will wait a few years, as long as we make this request clear to the spirit world. It's important that we let our kids be kids.

KNOW YOUR FRAME OF REFERENCE. When you are beginning to learn to interact more clearly with your guides and other beings in spirit form, it's helpful to know some of the ways these beings may try to communicate with you. Have you ever had an old memory, old song lyric, or even a fragrance from the past pop into your mind from out of nowhere? Well…sometimes that's them! Your guides and other spirits will often use your own memories, your own experiences, to convey their messages to you. Everything stored in your cell memory that you have ever felt, seen, heard, smelled, tasted, or experienced can be used. This frame of reference may include words, symbols, people, memories and past experiences, photos, songs, and song lyrics. Anything! For example, a medium is providing a reading and sees in her mind's eye the face of her own brother, whose name is Gerald. Her spirit guides or other spirit being may be showing her this because the name of the spirit being with whom she is communicating is also named Gerald. Or perhaps the spirit being is communicating that he is the brother of the person who is receiving the reading.

DEVELOP YOUR SYMBOL LIBRARY. As you learn and as you and your spirit guides use your frame of reference—your memories and experiences—to communicate, it may also be helpful to begin to develop your own symbol library. This is not a requirement, it's a personal choice. Not everyone chooses to develop a symbol library, but many find it can be helpful when receiving and conveying information, especially if they want to relay messages from spirit to other people. For example, if you want to build your symbol library, you can decide that when you are shown your brother Gerald, this means that either the name Gerald or a brother is significant. You can also designate certain symbols, like a caution sign that means that a person should avoid or be careful in a situation. A dove can mean at peace or a peaceful passing. A stop sign could be a symbol for you to stop giving a particular message to an individual, to alert you that perhaps it should be given to the person in a more private setting. Your symbol library will grow as quickly as you build it. The more symbols you can designate, the more tools you and your guides will have to communicate accurate and specific messages.

Strengthening Your Ability to Connect

In chapter 7, we focused on connecting with God and spirit in order to raise our vibration. To further develop our gift of intuition, and indeed to fulfill our soul's purpose, we want to add to these exercises to nurture and strengthen even further our connection with God, our higher selves, and the spirit world. This means opening and raising the vibration of our own energy, as well as working with spiritual beings and energies at a high vibration. And it means using additional exercises to learn to maintain this connection for longer and longer periods over time. And as we know, when we do this, we must also ensure balance by grounding, grounding, grounding.

First, prayer is a highly effective method that can help us strengthen our spiritual connection.

When we pray, this is our way of talking to God. Prayers can be anything you want them to be. Here are a few prayers that people have found helpful in opening to their gift of intuition:

> Dear God, I thank you for washing away all negativity in my spirit, mind, heart, and body, for filling me with your love and light. I pray that I may be opened to your Divine guidance and be pure in intention, motivation, thought, word, and deed in service to Your holy will.

> *Dear God, thank you for connecting me to your love and healing energy from both heaven and earth. Thank you for opening my heart to love, light, and the spiritual gifts you have entrusted to me. Thank you that I may fully open to and realize*

these gifts in fulfillment of my soul's purpose in your
Divine plan.

Dear God, thank you for this life, for this day,
and for the opportunity to use the gifts you have
given me to serve you in love and service to others.

I say yes to *God.*

Second, while prayer could be considered a form of talking to God, meditation is listening to God—and to our higher selves and other spiritual beings. Meditation serves to quiet our mind and allows us to simply be. Once in this state of being, we are also able to better connect with and communicate with our higher self and the spiritual realm.

When beginning to develop your spiritual gifts, I recommend starting with meditating for five, ten, or fifteen minutes at least three times a week. I advise that you do your surround, ground, and shield exercises first, followed by a brief breathing exercise (if it's not already included in the meditation itself), before you begin the meditation. The meditation itself could involve listening to an audio-guided meditation, or just sitting quietly with soft music and focusing on an image in your mind, like a candle flame, to quiet the mind. If you use an audio-guided meditation, you may find yourself listening and taking the journey word for word and then going off into your own imagination or experience. This is fine, as long as you have done your surround, ground, and shield exercises. As intrusive thoughts about your day, worries, or to-do list come up, do not focus on these or try to stop them. Simply put them in a bubble and let them float away.

Over time, as you continue to practice your meditation regularly, the number of intrusive thoughts will begin to decrease and you can gradually increase your meditation time. Try increasing the meditation by three to five minutes at first, and then continue to add three to five minutes as you become better and better at maintaining the connection.

There are many meditations that can help you learn to quiet your mind and connect spiritually.

While many of my own audio-guided meditations begin with a breathing exercise, some meditations may not. If you are using a meditation that does not include breathing, this simple breathing exercise can help you to relax and center yourself before you begin the meditation. Please do your surround, ground, and shield exercises first.

In choosing meditations to help you strengthen your ability to connect spiritually, I recommend starting with the

Breathing to Relax and Center Yourself*

- Sit or lie down in a comfortable position and close your eyes.
- Begin by breathing in through your nose, into your abdomen to the count of four.
- Hold your breath for four.
- And release, blowing the breath out your mouth for a count of four.
- And again, breathing in for four all the way into your belly.
- Hold it for four.
- And blow it out your mouth for four.
- And one last time, breathing in, all the way into your belly.
- Hold it for four.
- And blow it out your mouth for four.

---

* This breathing exercise can be used before a meditation, throughout the day if you feel you need to calm and center yourself, or in a circumstance where you are feeling anxious or in a panic mode.

Universal White Light Meditation (see chapter 5). This meditation will help you ground, heal and balance, and connect with spirit, all in one exercise.

Another important way to strengthen your ability to connect spiritually is to open yourself. You are actively looking to open yourself to and connect with a higher vibration of energy and to the entire Universe of love and light (with protection, of course). The meditation below, Breathing Through Your Chakras, for example, will help you to open, clear, and balance your chakras, thus also opening you to greater intuitive input. As always, please do your surround, ground, and shield exercises before beginning the meditation.

Breathing Through Your Chakras Meditation

The meditation you are about to experience is designed to help you open, clear, and balance your seven key chakras.

- → I would like you to begin by sitting in a comfortable space or perhaps lying down, and closing your eyes.
- → Begin by breathing in through your nose, into your abdomen, to the count of four.
- → Hold your breath for four.
- → Now release the breath, blowing it out your mouth for a count of four.
- → And again, breathe in, all the way into your belly.
- → Hold it for four.
- → And blow it out your mouth for four.

⇥ And one last time, breathing all the way in.

⇥ Hold it for four.

⇥ And blow it out your mouth for four.

⇥ Now I would like you to imagine that you are taking a breath through your crown chakra, located at the very top of your head.

⇥ Through your crown chakra, inhale for a count of four, breathing in God's white light. Imagine God's white light filling your crown chakra as you hold the breath for four, and then blow it out for four.

⇥ Take a deep breath for four. Hold it for four. And blow it out for four.

⇥ And now, imagine that you are taking a breath through the third-eye chakra, located in the center of your forehead or brow area.

⇥ Through your third-eye chakra, inhale for a count of four, breathing in God's white light. Imagine God's white light filling your third-eye chakra as you hold the breath for four, and then blow it out for four.

⇥ Again, breathe in for four... Hold it for four... And blow it out for four.

⇥ And now, imagine that you are taking a breath through the throat chakra, located in the center of your throat.

⇥ Through your throat chakra, inhale for a count of four, breathing in God's white light. Imagine God's white light filling your throat chakra as you hold the breath for four, and then blow it out for four.

⇥ Again, breathe in for four. Hold it... and blow it out for four.

⇁ And now, move to your heart chakra, located in the center of your chest.

⇁ Through your heart chakra, inhale for a count of four, breathing in God's white light. Imagine your heart and lungs filling with God's white light as you hold the breath for four, and then blow it out for four.

⇁ Again, breathe in for four, hold it...and blow it out for four.

⇁ Next, move to your solar plexus chakra, right below your rib cage or sternum.

⇁ Take a breath through your solar plexus. Inhale for four, breathing in God's white light. Imagine your solar plexus filling with God's white light as you hold the breath for four, and blow it out for four.

⇁ Breathe in for four. Hold it...blow it out.

⇁ And now, imagine that you are taking a breath through the sacral or spleen chakra, located just below and behind the naval.

⇁ Through your sacral or spleen chakra, inhale for a count of four, breathing in God's white light. Imagine God's white light filling your sacral chakra as you hold the breath for four, and then blow it out for four.

⇁ Again, breathe in for a count of four. Hold it for four, and blow it out for four.

⇁ Moving to the root chakra, located at the tailbone or base of your spine, imagine taking a breath through the root chakra. Inhale for four, breathing in God's white light. Imagine God's white light filling your root chakra as you hold the breath for four, and then blow it out.

> ⇝ Now imagine God's white light extending from your root chakra, deep into the earth, forming a ball of brilliant white light…and then, rising back up through your feet and spine, through your root, sacral, solar plexus, heart, throat, third-eye, and crown chakras…all the way back up to heaven, connecting and balancing you in the Divine energy of both heaven and earth.
>
> ⇝ And simply now…by closing your hands into a fist and slowly, gently opening your eyes, come back into the space where you began, knowing you are better for having done this.*

In using these prayers, meditations, and other exercises to open to and strengthen your ability to connect with your higher self, spiritual guides, and God, you are building the very foundation for developing your intuition and related spiritual gifts. In addition to the Universal White Light Meditation, there are many others, including those shared in chapters 5 and 7 and on my YouTube channel that will help you connect with spirit.

Enhancing Your Senses

Another way to help you build your intuitive muscle is to utilize visualizations or meditations that will increase your

---

* You can use this meditation as often as you wish to open, clear, and balance the seven main chakras.

awareness of your five human senses—and your ability to imagine or see, hear, taste, smell, and feel by thought. Learning to become aware of and experience our human senses by thought can result in strengthening and expanding our intuitive or "extrasensory" perceptions as well. But before beginning, you guessed it, please do your surround, ground, and shield exercises.

Experiencing Your Five Senses by Thought Meditation

The meditation you are about to experience is designed to help you become aware of your five senses, and your ability to experience them by thought or imagination.

- ⇁ Begin by sitting in a comfortable space or perhaps lying down, and closing your eyes.
- ⇁ And now, begin to breathe in through your nose to the count of four, holding it for four, and then blowing it out your mouth for four.
- ⇁ Again, take a breath in through your nose for a count of four, hold it for four, and blow it out your mouth for four.
- ⇁ Now imagine yourself going to your favorite beach, beginning to walk on the sand to find your place to lay down your blanket and settle in.
- ⇁ The sand feels warm under your feet. Are there many people on the beach at this moment?
- ⇁ Once you are settled, walk down to the shoreline, feel the warm, wet sand between your toes.

→ Step into the surf to feel the temperature of the water. How does it feel? Is the surf gently lapping the shore, or is the ocean rough today? Can you hear it? Can you hear the seagulls that are flying overhead? What kind of day is it? Is it sunny and hot? Are there white, puffy clouds in the sky? Or is the sky overcast?

→ Imagine now, that you are back at your blanket. You have brought some fruit along with you.

→ Take out your favorite fruit and smell it. Is it ripe and ready to eat? Or perhaps it's not quite the way you like it. Feel it, take a bite, taste it, enjoy it.

→ The day has gone way too fast and it's time to go home.

→ And simply now ... by closing your hands into a fist and slowly, gently opening your eyes, come back into the space where you began, knowing you are better for having done this.

Communicating with Spirit: Techniques to Manifest Your Intuitive Gift

As you continue to develop a closer connection and begin to try to communicate with or receive information from the Universe and the spirit world, it's important to pay attention to the different ways you can receive information and try different techniques to see what works for you. It's also important to practice, practice, practice. Before doing spiritual or intuitive work or exercises, always remember first to surround, ground, and shield in God's white light—and set your intention for the highest good.

First, as you go about your day-to-day life, begin to pay attention to your thoughts and your sensory perceptions. Recognize the still small voice within you. Take note of "random" thoughts, words, pictures, memories, songs, lyrics, or smells that may pop into your head. These random thoughts are often information that we are receiving from within—or from above (one and the same in my book). Keep a journal and document these insights as they occur.

Second, there are some simple exercises you can use to strengthen your intuitive muscles, and your ability to pick up information and energy connected to people, animals, objects, places, and the spirit world. These exercises will help you determine where your strengths are, but over time, also to improve your abilities to receive this energy and information psychically.

A few of these exercises:

- With a friend, have him or her place objects in an envelope and then try to intuit what those objects are. Try to be as detailed as possible.
- When talking to a friend on the phone, try to intuit detailed information such as what they are wearing, how their day went, or how their family is doing.
- Try holding an object in your hand and intuiting who owns it, where it's been, and whose energy might be connected to it (called psychometry). You can do this same thing by closing your eyes and holding a person's hand or a photograph. Is the person male or female? Child or adult? What do you see, hear, smell, taste, feel, or know from this object? Or with your eyes open or closed, what can you pick up about the

person or thing in the photograph? Who is it? Where
is it? What is the story behind this photograph?
- Place a deck of cards facedown on a table and fan
them out. Randomly select a card, still facing down,
and try to intuit what the card is. Is it red or black? Is
it a number card or face card? Is it a club, spade, heart,
or diamond? As you develop this intuitive muscle, you
may be able to determine the exact card that you have
selected.

For all of these exercises, do not overthink it. Just say or
write whatever pops into your head. Do not judge it or doubt
it, just say or write it. The more you practice, the better you
will get. Since there are multiple ways of communicating directly with beings in spirit form, there are multiple techniques
to help you assess and develop your abilities in this area. I'm
going to include just a few here, to help get you started in recognizing and developing your gifts.

DREAMS. Many of us—maybe even all of us—receive messages or visits from spiritual beings (including our loved
ones) while we are sleeping. For whatever reason, our conscious mind seems to be more quiet and our spiritual door
more open during this time. For many who are just starting
to pay attention to their intuition, this may be where they first
notice their gifts. There are several types of dreams, two of
which are precognitive and visitation dreams. In precognitive
dreams, we may see, hear, or otherwise come to know information that is predictive of events in the future. Some people
will have these dreams over and over again until they come
true. These are often positive dreams but, in some cases, they
can be negative, foretelling plane crashes, catastrophic
weather, and deaths. I advise people who are having dreams

that are foretelling negative events to ask their spirit guides, "Please do not show me negative information or events, unless there is a way for me to help prevent them or bring help or healing in some way."

Another kind of dream is the visitation dream. Many people visit with their loved ones in their sleep. They may see them, hear them, or feel them. Some people see faces or see or hear words, as they are falling asleep or waking up. Some, like MaryAnn, experience short or even prolonged discussions with a loved one while in a dream state. Sometimes, people may wake up and simply feel like they were with their loved one, or that their loved one was here.

For this reason, I highly recommend that you take a notepad to bed with you and write down any dreams you have or messages you may get. In fact, you can even ask God, your spirit guides, or a loved one a question before you go to sleep and see if you wake up with an answer! Once you become more aware of and acknowledge these connections and messages, they often will make their way into the daylight hours as well.

MEDITATION. As we noted earlier, meditation is an excellent way to build your ability or capacity to connect—and an effective way to "listen." Similar to receiving messages or visits during sleep, many people who are just learning about their intuitive gifts will begin to notice this happening during meditation. While receiving messages during meditation alone is not ideal for a professional psychic or medium, it can be an effective gateway to recognizing and developing your gifts further. To help my clients and students get started, I often recommend trying a simple meditation such as "A Journey to Visit Your Loved Ones Through Meditation." Remember: surround-ground-shield first.

A Journey to Visit Your Loved Ones through Meditation

This meditation is designed to allow you to visit with a loved one who has crossed over to the other side. Know that spirit is with us and around us whenever we think about them and that your imagination is the bridge to spirit.

⇁ I would like you to sit quietly now in a comfortable position, close your eyes, and begin to breathe in through your nose to the count of four. Hold it for four…and now blow it out your mouth for four.

⇁ Please repeat. Breathing all the way into your abdomen…hold it…and blowing it all the way out your mouth.

⇁ I would like you now to visualize or imagine yourself surrounded in a beautiful, translucent bubble of God's white light and protection.

⇁ And to ground yourself now in God's light, by imagining three cords of white light, one attached to the bottom of each of your feet and one coming from your tailbone.

⇁ Imagine these three cords of light shooting through the floor and all the way into the earth, locking you into the earth like the roots of a tree…Continuing to breathe slowly and more regular now, so relaxed, so serene, and so calm.

⇁ Now I would like you to picture or imagine that you are in a beautiful garden filled with flowers of every color, plants, trees and green grass.

- ⇀ There are many places to rest in the garden, perhaps on a bench, or under a big old tree, or sitting on a large rock beside a stream. Look around and find a place to sit and rest.
- ⇀ Put out the thought that you would like to meet with your loved one that has left the physical world.
- ⇀ Sit quietly for a moment and begin to feel or imagine your loved one coming toward you and sitting down next to you.
- ⇀ Your loved one is happy, healthy, and whole. There is no pain, no sickness, no fear on the other side—only peace, joy, and love.
- ⇀ Embrace him or her and take a moment to feel and absorb the energy that is connected to your loved one.
- ⇀ You may ask a question if you wish or just sit quietly and enjoy the feelings of love and happiness that your loved one is sending to you.
- ⇀ You can communicate simply by thoughts and feelings.
- ⇀ Listen for or feel the answer.
- ⇀ If you do not receive an answer at this moment, be patient and know that it will come eventually.
- ⇀ Your loved ones continue to send you signs all of the time in the physical world. Through a song, a paragraph in a book, a scene in a movie. Perhaps through a colorful bird that keeps showing up, or sending you pennies or dimes that simply appear out of nowhere. Allow yourself to be open to see, feel, or hear them.
- ⇀ All things are possible with time and patience.

- → Spend a few more moments sitting with your loved one now, as soon it will be time for you to leave the garden.
- → It is time now to say good-bye and thank your loved one for this brief visit and know that you can always return to the garden whenever you wish.
- → You have the ability to communicate with your loved ones anytime your heart desires.
- → And simply now by closing your hands into a fist, slowly and gently opening your eyes, come back into the space where you began.*

Do not be concerned if this meditation does not result in your recognizing a visit with a loved one right away. Just keep practicing, and the more you do, the more information you will begin to receive. Be patient with yourself; it will come.

FOCUSED ACTIVITY. Many professional psychics and mediums use an activity that helps them to focus their conscious minds, to get into "the zone" in order to connect with and bring in spiritual information or energy more effectively. I think of this almost as a form of meditation, as it seems to clear the mind of clutter and open it to other realms. Some people may begin their messages by scribbling—making huge doodles or crazy markings that appear to mean nothing at all. Others will write random words, like a person's name or a

---

* This meditation can be done as often as you wish. This guided meditation can be found on "Guided Meditations with Pat Longo" on iTunes, Amazon, and other digital platforms.

word or phrase that may stand out to them in the information they are receiving. Others may use angel cards, tarot cards, or another type of device to help facilitate their communication. You can try all of these techniques. Simply ask God, your spirit guides, angels, or other beings a question. Then try the scribbling, angel cards, tarot cards, or other method of your choice and see what happens.

AUTOMATIC WRITING. Similarly, many people like to start to receive messages with what's called "automatic writing." This is where you simply put pen or pencil to paper and let the messages come. You don't think, you just write. Some people will receive beautiful, elegant writings from Divine beings—even messages for humanity. Some will receive letters from their spirit guides or from loved ones. Others receive poems and rhymes. Often, this writing is done rapidly and it may appear in a handwriting that is not your own. The important thing here is to put the pen right to the paper. Do not wait to hear and figure out the message before you begin writing. Don't wait, just write.

In addition, if you are going along, minding your business one day and begin experiencing a sense of urgency or restlessness, or you begin hearing, seeing, or feeling the same words or message playing in your mind over and over again, this may mean that an automatic writing is in the wings. This is exactly what happened to Steven. If this happens, find a notepad and start writing. Just put the pen to paper and let it flow.

In the meantime, a good way to get started with automatic writing is simply to ask for one. (See the box on p. 212.)

You can try this exercise, asking questions of God, your spirit guides, angels, loved ones, or whomever you wish. The more you practice, the more you will receive. Importantly, if you start experiencing the urge or need to do automatic

Practicing Communication with Automatic Writing

- Find a quiet room where you will not be disturbed.
- Do your surround, ground, and shield exercises before you begin (chapter 5).
- Ask God, your spirit guides, and angels to be with you and light a white candle.
- Then put your pen to the paper and ask a question, such as "Dear Spirit Guide, what would you like to teach me today?" or "Dear Angels, what message would you like to give me today?"
- Then let your pen do the work. Do not think. Do not interpret. Do not judge. Do not wait. Just write.

writing frequently, or for long periods of time, you need to set boundaries. Using your thoughts, you need to tell your spirit guides and the spirit world when you are available for communicating. Be sure to tell them in earth time (such as Mondays through Fridays, 7:00 p.m. to 8:00 p.m. eastern standard time, earth time). Like any other form of communication, you also need to make it clear who is and who is not permitted to send messages. I have known very gifted people whose lives became overwhelmed by automatic writing, becoming completely consumed, penning for hours and days at a time. The writings were beautiful, but the Universe is endless and one person cannot write it all. This is not a balanced, healthy way to live or to be of service to yourself or anyone else. Set those boundaries.

PSYCHOMETRY. This technique involves the holding of an object, photo, or even someone's hand to communicate with an energy that's associated with the object. Just like this method can be used to pick up energy and information psychically, it can also be used to communicate directly with a being in spirit form. For example, you may wish to hold a person's photo or item of jewelry to help facilitate the connection with that being in the spirit world.

PHYSICAL MOVEMENT. Many people find that some type of physical movement can help the flow of spiritual or intuitive energy. Although walking is not an ideal technique for a professional intuitive who is providing a one-on-one reading to a client, it can be a good way for some people to get started in manifesting their intuitive gifts—and ultimately can also work well for those who are reading in front of a group of people. If you feel anxious, jittery, or restless energy as you begin trying to connect and communicate, you can try walking to help you move the energy. In the beginning, just walk around your house, in the park, or other area and think of a person or situation and see what information you receive. If this works for you, you may also like to try more subtle ways to help move the energy. Many people use activities such as rubbing their hands together, tapping their fingers, shaking their hands a bit, or rocking back and forth.

I recommend that you try all of these techniques, and practice, practice, practice. See what works for you. Oftentimes, people will start out using one or more techniques and will outgrow them and graduate to others as their gift strengthens.

Ask and You Shall Receive

Over time, as you designate time to connect with spirit and practice these different techniques, your connection and abilities will strengthen and you may begin to receive more information. This information may include messages to help and guide you and your loved ones. For some of you, it may also include messages for other people. As this begins to happen more, there are a few tips that will help you in delivering a message that is as accurate, specific, and complete as possible. One of the most important points is to begin to ask for more information. If you ask, you shall receive.

INTERPRET AND VALIDATE. This process comes into play once you feel your intuitive skills are progressing and you begin to receive messages not only for you, but for other people as well. While our guides or other beings in spirit form are utilizing our frame of reference and symbol library to communicate with us, it is our job to interpret and validate the messages. This is done in collaboration with spirit and with the person for whom the message is intended, as he or she will need to validate the information you are providing.

In general, beings in spirit form must work to lower their vibration in order to communicate with those of us on earth, just as we are raising our vibration to communicate with them. In doing this, they often will seek to be efficient and will not waste energy. They will tell us only what is needed, and it's our job to ask the necessary follow-up questions and to work with the "client" to validate the information.

For example, many years ago, I decided to treat myself to a much needed afternoon nap. I was all settled in on the couch and just drifting off to sleep, when I suddenly saw an image of a calendar flash before my mind's eye. It appeared and vanished so quickly that I didn't see much, but I did manage to make out that the month started with a J and that there was a date highlighted in yellow on the upper right-hand corner of the page. Now awake, I acknowledged my spirit guides,

"Thank you, I see it's a calendar with a month starting with a J. What else do you want me to know?" I then saw in my mind's eye a little American flag. So I again thanked my guides and asked them, "I see the flag so I know it is Memorial day, Veteran's day, the Fourth of July, or Labor Day. Which date are you showing me? I then saw a flash of red, white, and blue fireworks, and I knew my guides were showing me the Fourth of July. So I thanked them, acknowledged the date, and asked them what else they wanted to tell me. I then saw an image of my daughter Christine as a small infant. Christine, who was now 28, was pregnant and her baby was due on July 5th. In seeing this image of her as an infant, I recognized that this message was about Christine and her baby. I then felt immediately that her baby would be coming early. At that time, the phone rang and I had to answer it, so my intuitive session ended. As it turns out, my daughter went into labor over 2 weeks early, on June 19th. Now, I do not consider myself a medium, but everyone possesses an ability to communicate with the spirit world—and it can start with baby steps such as these. In this example, had I not noticed the message and asked a follow-up question, I would simply have seen a vague and fleeting image of a calendar page. I would not have realized it had anything to do with my daughter and the baby who was coming (sooner than we thought). The important thing is for us to recognize these visual flashes (whether they be calendars, people, memories, words); voices or sounds; and feelings as the messages that they are—and to thank our guides, validate the message, and ask the questions needed to receive the full message.

When receiving and relaying a message, all messages are important. But as our skills become stronger, we want to learn to hold the energy and ask the needed questions to validate the information with the recipient and, from spirit, gain more helpful details. So as you are learning, you will first just be trying to open, connect, and receive. But as you begin to communicate more, remember to ask questions and then listen for the answers. You can do this when receiving information in conscious thought, in meditation, and even in your dreams.

ASK FOR DETAILS. When you begin working to become aware of and develop your ability to receive and understand intuitive messages from the spirit world, you want to connect, listen, and write down or otherwise note the information you receive. As your abilities strengthen and you begin to receive messages for yourself and others, it's important to be able to convey tangible details to demonstrate the validity of the connection. This is why we will often see a highly gifted medium begin by describing how a loved one passed or with information that only this person and the client would know. This detailed information does two things. First, it validates for the recipient that this is their loved one. Second, it demonstrates for the recipient that your gift is genuine. As your abilities progress, I recommend this approach, asking to be given detailed information early on, so that it will be clear that the rest of the message (for example, I am okay, I am at peace, I love you) is also genuine. While there are many highly gifted individuals providing messages with integrity and accuracy, there are also many with less ability or lacking in integrity, seeking to take advantage of vulnerable people in vulnerable situations. The details-first approach will help the client make this distinction and avoid being exploited by those who are ill-intended or misguided. With the reinforcement of such details, he or she can fully accept the message and the healing that comes with it.

PRACTICE, PRACTICE, PRACTICE. When you feel ready, you can begin practicing your psychic or mediumship skills with individual readings for "friends of friends" whom you do not know. Over time, as you are able to validate a high percentage of the information you have been receiving, you may wish to start practicing group readings. To do this, you can ask friends to organize small groups of their friends, whom you don't know, for you to read. In the beginning, I strongly advise that you give your messages while sitting or standing with your back to a wall. This is easier at the start, as messages often can seem to come from every direction when positioned in the center of the room and this can be confusing. Always begin by setting your intention and surrounding, grounding, and shielding. Before you start, ask your spirit guides for clarity, efficiency, and speed with the purpose of delivering constructive messages meant to bring love and healing. Remind them that you do not wish to see negative events, unless you can help to prevent or heal them. Use a symbol, such as lighting a white candle, to let the spirit realm know you are ready to start the session. Finally, as you continue to practice, remember that the goal is not to become a professional psychic or medium. The goal is to discover and develop your intuitive abilities, whatever they may be, to help guide you and your loved ones in fulfilling your soul's purpose and living your best life. For some of you, that may mean a future as a professional in this area. For most of you, it will be another amazing destiny. It's all about opening to your unique gifts and living your truth.

The steps in this book are meant to get you started on the path to discovering and developing your gift of intuition—and to help you reduce or even eliminate spiritually based anxiety and related symptoms. I recommend finding a credible spiritual teacher or mentor who can help guide you in continuing to develop your spiritual gifts, including those of a psychic, mediumship, and spiritual healing nature. There may be spiritual teachers in your community who are known for their integrity and good works. You can also take advantage of other books as well as seminars, workshops, and classes offered in-person or via webinar or other online venue. For a listing of resources to help guide you in your journey, see the appendix: "More Tools and Resources."

And remember, everyone's gifts are different. We all have intuition, we all have the ability to connect and communicate. But we all perceive and receive it differently. The information may come through mediumship or more general psychic abilities. It may come through with one technique and not another. See where your strengths lie and what works for you. And don't worry if you don't receive the answers or communications immediately on-demand. I hear many stories of people receiving messages in the shower! Just keep doing the work and pay attention to the signs around you, and to the thoughts you are having throughout the day.

As your gifts strengthen and as you begin to receive more and more intuitive guidance for yourself and others, it's important to maintain your daily homework to protect and maintain your own healthy, balanced state of being. It's important to continue to love and honor yourself—and always, to share your gift with integrity...and with love.

CHAPTER 11

It's All About Love

OVER TWENTY YEARS AGO, THE realization that I had been given the gift of spiritual healing came to me as a surprise, even a shock. Yet, as my gift continued to develop, I felt more and more like me. I remember vividly praying to God and asking that those in need of healing be placed in my path. I wanted desperately to learn more, to develop my gift further, to be the best healer I could be. I committed to striving to be a clear channel for God's love, light, and healing energy.

When I asked God for guidance in this journey, I intuitively received one strong, unmistakable message. The message was: "Open your heart and everything else will follow."

Open your heart. This sounded so simple, but what did it mean? I wondered—and then, deep down, I felt it. I knew. It meant that I needed to let go of anything that was keeping my heart closed, walled off, or in fragments. I needed to live from my whole heart, not pieces of it. It meant that I needed to begin to see myself and others through the eyes of love, empathy, and compassion. To live without judgment. To forgive more. To love more. To love all. As I was promised, as I learned to do this more fully, my gift of healing continued to develop and more and more people in need were placed in my path. I believe the purpose of our spiritual gifts, and indeed the purpose of our lives, is to learn to receive and to give love, to evolve to the very consciousness of love.

As you continue on your journey to develop your spiritual gifts, it's important to share your gifts with love. Just as I believe *healing* is the process of bringing one's spirit, mind, heart, and physical body into balance in love—I believe psychic, mediumship, and other intuitive gifts should be used to connect with love, to communicate love, to forgive, and to heal.

When you are ready to begin to use and share your gifts, these important steps will help you connect and communicate that energy of love and healing:

Set Your Intention

In sharing our psychic and mediumship abilities, the purpose of receiving and delivering messages from the Universe and spiritual realm is to receive and deliver only constructive messages that offer the opportunity for healing or the prevention of suffering. We should set our intention before beginning our spiritual work for the day to receive messages or provide healing for the highest good, in God's love and light. We need to clearly indicate that we do *not* wish to see death or negative events that we cannot stop, prevent, or otherwise bring healing to. Similarly, the intention when working as a spiritual healer is to serve as a vessel or channel to bring God's love, light, and healing energy to the recipient, for his or her highest good.

Ask Permission

When sharing our intuitive messages, it's important that we ask permission from the recipient before we do so. We don't want to ambush people with a message, we don't want to embarrass anyone in front of others, and we don't want to deliver a message in a way that may be counterproductive to our purpose of providing healing. Similarly, spiritual healers should not walk up to people and tell them about their illnesses, or put their hands on people without asking first. Healers can send healing energy by thought, which I encourage. This can be done without verbal notice, and without being invasive or intrusive. However, even when sending healing by thought we should ask that the healing be sent "in alignment with the will of God and the will of the individual." This way, the energy is offered respectfully and, if it is not wanted, it will not be received.

Deliver, Don't Read

Our job is to deliver the mail, not to read the mail. As noted earlier, this means that there is no place for EGO in our spiritual work. The message is not our own; we do not judge, doubt, or fear the message. In another example from my early days in Holly's class, I remember the first intuitive message I was able to give. Holly asked us each to tune in to our intuition to give a message or information to someone else in the class. So I turned to the woman next to me, and I asked my spirit guides to help me receive a message for her. I was trying my best, but all I saw was this bizarre image of a court jester. I saw him in his little hat, pointy shoes, the bells and the whole thing. I was trying so hard to tune in, and this is what I got. A court jester.

Holly asked me to convey what I received, but I couldn't, I felt ridiculous. "They will think I'm stark raving mad," I thought to myself. But Holly insisted, explaining that it was not my job to judge what I receive, just to receive and to deliver. So reluctantly I said to the woman, "I see a court jester with a little hat, pointy shoes, and bells." Well, the woman gasped out loud. She was astounded, not because she thought I was crazy, but because she had just finished making a court jester costume for her son for his upcoming school play. So this information, while I doubted it and felt foolish in delivering it, was actually completely accurate and highly specific and validating to this particular lady. It isn't our job to judge ourselves or the messages that we are giving, but to have faith and deliver them as gracefully and gently as we can.

Deliver, Don't Throw

We don't read the mail, nor do we throw the mail. In delivering a message, not only should we not judge or doubt, but we should seek to deliver the message as gently as possible—with grace and with the intention to bring love and healing. We should not deliver a message in a way that will be jarring or upsetting to the recipient. We should not be focusing on how we, as the messenger, will look the most impressive in delivering the message. We are not aiming for drama. We are using our words, our voice, our energy (and those of spirit) to bring love and healing.

Maintain Confidentiality

This is important whether we are "just practicing," providing services free of charge, or maintaining a professional psychic, medium, or healer practice. Just like when we visit a physician's office, a psychic, medium, or healer should keep confidential the identity of a client and the content of a client's visit. We should not tell others that so-and-so came to visit me, or did you hear this woman is ill? This is true even when we are helping multiple members of one family or helping friends who know each other. We cannot assume others are privy to the information that is shared with us or with the information we have shared with one member of a family or group in a private session. In the same way, it is also important to be sensitive about the type of information you convey in a group or public setting. Anything that could be sensitive should be shared later, in private not public. This type of confidentiality is essential to providing a space and experience that is safe—and healing.

Give Back

For those of you who wish to use your gifts professionally, you are entitled to abundance in love, light, and yes, finances. Like anyone, you need to make a living. When you are just starting out and doing the "practice" readings, I advise that you do not charge for these sessions. This is a mutually beneficial arrangement, wherein the clients are receiving helpful messages and you are being assisted in developing your gifts. I recommend that you continue to do practice sessions for as long as needed, until you are consistently providing readings that are clear, detailed, able to be validated, and healing. Once you have been able to do this and are starting your life as a professional in this area, you are entitled to charge for your services. You are not charging for your gift. Just like a plumber or any other professional who provides a service, you are charging for your time, energy, and experience. However, as part of our commitment to integrity and intention to love and serve the highest good, I advise my students that clients should not come for healings in an unnecessary or excessive manner. Some clients with chronic or advanced dis-ease may need ongoing sessions and support. But if a client is feeling better and doing well, he or she can use their homework instructions to maintain his or her own health and may not need ongoing maintenance sessions. Similarly, if someone is requesting frequent intuitive readings and appears to be reliant on this to make life decisions, or always wants to know the future, this is not a balanced, healthy form of seeking guidance. And finally, I believe it's important to find a way to give back, perhaps making a few sessions a year available to people who cannot afford them or offering your services to a charitable cause on occasion. I do not recommend that you do this to the extent of abusing yourself. It needs to be done in a way that is balanced, maintains healthy boundaries, and feels right to you. But if our purpose is to love and serve, then our intention must be to make this love and healing accessible to as many people as possible, not only to a privileged few. This is a truth that I believe applies to all spiritual gifts, including psychic, mediumship, healing, and teaching work.

Remember: Honor Thyself

Just as we strive to use our gifts to bring healing and love to others, it's important to remember to love ourselves. Part of loving ourselves is making sure we maintain our own healing and health on an ongoing basis, to ensure that we are living, learning, and sharing our gifts with—you guessed it—balance.

Have I said a hundred times yet that healing is all a big balancing act? Balance brings healing. Healing brings balance. Balance is important for everyone, and especially those who are developing their intuition and doing spiritual work. All of the instructions and exercises we have discussed so far will help you maintain your healing and balance. You will need balance in your daily life (honoring yourself). You will need balance in your communication with the spirit world (setting boundaries). You will need surrounding, grounding, and shielding to provide protection and balance with your connection with other energies, including those of the spirit world. You will need to identify, forgive, and let go of old hurts to free yourself emotionally. You will need to set aside EGO. And you will need to work diligently to keep an energy balance in your four bodies, your chakras, and your whole self. It is staying in balance that allows the energy, the life force, to flow. Balance will ensure that your gifts are strong and are being used in a way that is safe and healing for yourself and others.

In addition to the other tools in this book, you may find this meditation—Balancing Your Energy Centers Meditation—helpful in keeping yourself balanced, clear, and in the flow of God's universal energy and life force as you continue to discover and develop your intuitive gifts. Please be sure to surround, ground, and shield first, as always.

Balancing Your Energy Centers Meditation

The meditation you are about to experience is designed to help you balance the energy centers in your body.

- ↝ I would like you to begin by sitting in a comfortable space, or perhaps lying down.
- ↝ Simply now, begin by closing your eyes, breathing in through your nose to the count of four, holding it for a count of four, and blowing it out your mouth for four.
- ↝ Repeat it, breathing in for four, holding it for four, and blowing it out your mouth for four.
- ↝ Imagine yourself soaring through the sky like a bird, free to be who or whatever you desire.
- ↝ Envision a rainbow up ahead, the colors so vivid and bright.
- ↝ Head toward the red end of the rainbow.
- ↝ Feel the color, as it increases your stamina and endurance.
- ↝ As you slowly soar through it, taking it all in.
- ↝ And now, you find yourself flooded with the freshness of the bright orange light of the rainbow.
- ↝ Absorbing it into your body like a thousand freshly squeezed oranges, supplying you with strength and vitality.
- ↝ You have now reached the yellow spectrum of the rainbow.
- ↝ Imagine you are enfolded in the warm rays of the sun, and a feeling of purity and love fills and surrounds you.
- ↝ Gradually you move into the green ray of the rainbow.
- ↝ Breathing it in, filling yourself with healing and harmony.
- ↝ The magnificence of the sky blue ray has now approached.

⇀ Breathe it into the pores of your skin, quieting your mind and calming your thoughts.

⇀ The deep indigo ray blankets you now, and you begin to feel lighter and lighter, with a sense of serenity and peace.

⇀ Finally, you are soaring through the violet purple rays of the rainbow, feeling a deep tranquility in your soul, at one with your maker.

⇀ Simply now, by closing your hands into a fist and slowly opening your eyes, come back into the space where you began, knowing you are better for having done this.*

In addition to doing your daily homework to maintain a healthy state of balance, it's important to know that individuals with extreme empath-related sensitivity and intuitive gifts can, at times, experience breakthrough symptoms such as anxiety, headache, nausea, or taking on or feeling the emotional or physical pain of others. The three tools below may help you in managing these symptoms if and when they occur:

- If you do experience an anxiety or panic attack, use a breathing technique to breathe your way through it (chapter 9). Inhale through your nose to a count of four, hold it for four, and exhale out your mouth to a count of four. Be sure to take deep breaths into your belly, rather than short, shallow breaths into your

---

* This meditation can be done as often as needed. This guided meditation can be found on my YouTube channel at www.youtube.com/user/thepatlongochannel.

chest. Focus on your breathing, and breathe your way out of the panic. It isn't about thinking, it's about breathing. When the panic resolves, be sure to re-apply your surround, ground, and shield exercises (chapter 5).

• If you experience frequent headaches, this may be due to excess spiritual energy coming in through your crown and third-eye chakras. In some people, this pain can also extend to neck and shoulder area. To prevent and treat this, imagine that in each of your ears is an air release, like you would see on a bicycle tire. Imagine that you are "letting out the air" from your head through both of your ears. Do this for ten seconds each night before bed, whether you have a headache at the time or not. It will help to minimize the number and severity of spiritually related headaches that you experience. If you have an active headache, use this same exercise to help dissipate the pain, then repeat on a daily basis for maintenance.

• If you are suddenly, inexplicably feeling a change in your mood, feeling emotionally sad or erratic for no reason, or feeling unexplained physical pain, you may be feeling the spiritual, mental, emotional, or physical pain of others. If you experience this, say silently or out loud: "Be gone. You are not of me." Say it three times. If this works to alleviate the emotional distur-bance or physical pain, then you know it was not yours. Please also be sure to reapply the surround, ground, and shield exercises at that time.

As we learn to maintain our own health and balance, and as we continue to discover and develop our own gifts of intu-ition, it's important to be open to whatever that inner voice, that inner sense of knowing, whispers to us. For many of us, a strong sense of intuition will enrich and enhance our lives, guiding us to be the very best parent, friend, or neighbor possible, or painter, musician, teacher, homemaker, physician, nurse, engineer, or other profession. Our intuition will lead and guide us in fulfilling our own soul's purpose on this earth. And we don't always know what that will be! For me, part of my journey in loving myself and listening to my inner voice, was to start saying no to the things I didn't want, and take up dancing and bowling lessons. Believe me, I will never be a professional dancer or bowler, but when I made the decision to make time for me, this is when a whole new world opened up for me. In listening to and loving myself and taking those bowling and dance lessons a couple of nights a week, my intuitive gifts began to emerge and ultimately led to my becoming a professional spiritual healer and teacher. Whatever path is ours, these gifts are of God and they are a part of us, to develop and to share to bring healing and love to our own lives and to others.

And oh what an amazing and miraculous love we can bring! Just think how many hearts we can open, how many spirits we can lift, how much light we can shine with the simple courage to be ourselves and the mindful intention to love.

In writing this book, my intention is to bring that love to you—to serve as a channel of God's love and light, to provide you with the healing you need for your highest good, for your highest love. Today, I ask you to open your heart to participate in and receive this gift of love and healing. Open your heart... and everything else will follow.

To receive it. To give it. To be it.

It's all about love...

More Tools and Resources

You are on your way! It is my hope that you will move forward with this book as your tool kit, utilizing the guidance and simple spiritual tools provided to help you care for your spiritual self: protecting your energy, finding healing and balance, beginning to open to your intuition and other related spiritual gifts, and in doing so, eliminating the spiritual causes of anxiety and other suffering in your life. Indeed, these spiritual healing steps are meant to heal and to restore and maintain your balance in spirit-mind-heart-body. As such, they will help not only those of you with anxiety, but those who are struggling with other symptoms and dis-ease—and those who simply want to stay healthy, balanced, and whole. So too, the exercises provided to help you discover and develop your intuition will be helpful not only to those of you with anxiety, but to everyone. After all, we all have a gift of intuition to guide us on our earthly journey.

In continuing on your spiritual path, I highly recommend that you seek out credible, trusted spiritual teachers, mentors, and authors to guide you along the way. There are many, many wonderful spiritual teachers who are dedicated to this work—

and with the digital technology of today, they are highly accessible online, if not in person. Just a small note of caution: There are also those who offer spiritual teaching or other services who are misinformed, misguided, or even fraudulent. So whether it be for classes, meditations, courses, or other opportunities, please be careful to ensure that the spiritual teacher or mentor is coming from a place of knowledge, integrity, and the intention for the highest good.

I have included below a list of additional resources to get you started. These resources include a few of the authors, teachers, and information I trust. May your journey be blessed with love, with love, with love; with light, with light, with light; to heal, to heal, to heal.

Suggested Reading

ECHO BODINE
> A Still, Small Voice: A Psychic's Guide to Awakening Intuition
> Echoes of the Soul

THERESA CAPUTO
> There's More to Life Than This: Healing Messages, Remarkable Stories, and Insight About the Other Side from the Long Island Medium
> You Can't Make This Stuff Up: Life-Changing Lessons from Heaven
> Good Grief: Heal Your Soul, Honor Your Loved Ones, and Learn to Live Again

MARYANN DIMARCO
> Believe, Ask, Act: Divine Steps to Raise Your Intuition, Create Change, and Discover Happiness

WAYNE DYER
The Power of Intention

SHAKTI GAWAIN
Creative Visualization

ESTHER AND JERRY HICKS
Ask and It Is Given: Learning to Manifest Your Desires

LAURA LYNNE JACKSON
The Light Between Us: Stories from Heaven, Lessons for the Living
Signs: The Secret Language of the Universe

MARY C. NEAL
To Heaven and Back

KIM RUSSO
The Happy Medium: Life Lessons from the Other Side
Your Soul Purpose: Learn How to Access the Light Within

FLORENCE SCOVEL SHINN
The Wisdom of Florence Scovel Shinn

ROBIN SHARMA
The Monk Who Sold His Ferrari
Who Will Cry When You Die?

Helpful Meditations

PAT LONGO
Guided Meditations with Pat Longo: On iTunes, Amazon, and other digital platforms; *other meditations:* Pat Longo Channel on YouTube, www.youtube.com/

OPRAH AND DEEPAK
 21-Day Meditation Experience (and others), chopracenter-meditation.com.

MAUREEN GARTH
 Moonbeam: A Book of Meditations for Children
 Starbright: Meditations for Children
 Sunshine: More Meditations for Children
 Earthlight: New Meditations for Children
 The Inner Garden: Meditations for Life from 9 to 90

Seminars, Workshops, and Events

Please visit my website, patlongo.net, and social media sites to find more tools and resources, news, and information on upcoming seminars, workshops, and events.